*Mosby's*
# CURBSIDE CLINICIAN
## INFECTIOUS DISEASES

# *Mosby's*
# CURBSIDE CLINICIAN
## INFECTIOUS DISEASES

FARRIN A. MANIAN, MD, MPH
Chief, Division of Infectious Diseases
St. John's Mercy Medical Center
St. Louis, Missouri

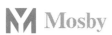 Mosby

St. Louis  Baltimore  Boston  Carlsbad  Chicago  Minneapolis  New York  Philadelphia  Portland
London  Milan  Sydney  Tokyo  Toronto

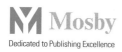

Dedicated to Publishing Excellence

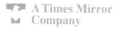

A Times Mirror
Company

Executive Editor: Michael J. Brown
Developmental Editor: Laura C. Berendson
Project Manager: Patricia Tannian
Project Specialist: Suzanne C. Fannin
Composition Specialist: Terri Knapp
Book Design Manager: Gail Morey Hudson
Manufacturing Manager: Dave Graybill
Cover Designer: Teresa Breckwoldt

Printed in the United States of America
Composition by Mosby Electronic Production, St. Louis
Printing/binding by R.R. Donnelley & Sons Company

Mosby–Year Book, Inc.
11830 Westline Industrial Drive
St. Louis, Missouri 63146

**International Standard Book Number 0-8151-2345-0**

97 98 99 00 01 / 9 8 7 6 5 4 3 2 1

*To my children*
**Josh, Jami, Jennifer,** *and* **CJ**

*It is noble to seek truth, and it is beautiful to find it. It is the ancient feeling of the human heart—that knowledge is better than riches; and it is deeply and sacredly true.*

**Sydney Smith**

*Any piece of knowledge I acquire today has a value at this moment exactly proportioned to my skill to deal with it. Tomorrow, when I know more, I recall that piece of knowledge and use it better.*

**Mark Van Doren**

# Preface

In the course of caring for our patients, we never cease to learn from them. We also learn a great deal from our colleagues who often informally help us manage patients by responding to our "curbside questions." Indeed, questions such as "Can I pick your brain?" or "Can I curbside you for a minute?" are well familiar to many of us, reflecting our need for a readily accessible and most up-to-date knowledge source. When carefully studied and tabulated, these questions should help identify topics and specific clinical situations important to physicians practicing in the "real world."

The *Mosby's Curbside Clinician: Infectious Diseases* is the culmination of work that began in 1990, when I started to record and catalog all curbside questions directed to me as an infectious disease physician practicing in a community hospital in St. Louis, Missouri. With the help of my colleague, Dr. David McKinsey, who has a similar practice in Kansas City, Missouri, I was able to study over 2000 such questions and identified the most frequently asked topics and questions (*Clin Infect Dis* 22:303-307, 1996), which serve as the basis of this book. Thus the topics selected for *Mosby's Curbside Clinician: Infectious Diseases* are based on actual questions asked by clinicians working in the "trenches." In addition to listing the most frequently asked questions and providing a response with selected up-to-date references, this book also lists many stimulating and challenging questions to which even the consultant may not have a ready answer and has to search the literature.

The MedLine service of the National Library of Congress was used extensively to access the most current published literature before a response was formulated. Often the response provided is a mosaic of two or more referenced articles or works synthesized by the author for the sake of conciseness and clarity. Whenever possible, the reader should refer to the pertinent articles or textbooks listed for more complete understanding of the subject matter in question.

There are several caveats. This book is not intended to replace appropriate formal consultations on specific patients. The clinician should use his or her judgment regarding the appropriateness of informal consultations; related guidelines on this subject have been previously published (*JAMA* 275:145-147, 1996). Moreover, as new information is constantly published, the answers to some questions may not necessarily be the most up-to-date at the time the information is sought. Lastly, as errors may still occur in the course of preparing the manuscript, when there is doubt, the reader is encouraged to verify the response independently.

I hope that you find *Mosby's Curbside Clinician: Infectious Diseases* useful and practical. Writing this book has enhanced my knowledge of many infectious disease conditions, and I hope that it will do the same for you. Comments and suggestions for future editions are appreciated.

**Farrin A. Manian**

## ACKNOWLEDGMENTS

The author thanks Ms. Tammy Gillman for her generous and unrelenting support of this book; Mr. Emil St. Pellicer for enduring hours of data entry and editing; David S. McKinsey, M.D., for recording many of the questions; the staff of St. John's Mercy Medical Library for their timely retrieval of journal articles; and the medical staff and housestaff at St. John's Mercy Medical Center, whose thoughtful and stimulating questions were the prime catalyst for publication of this book.

# Contents

## Cellulitis

## Ciprofloxacin

## Herpes Simplex Virus

## Herpes Zoster

## Human Immunodeficiency Virus

## Lower Respiratory Tract Infections

## Lyme Disease

## Malaria Prophylaxis

## Meningitis

## Urinary Tract Infections

## Vancomycin

## Varicella (Chicken Pox)

## Index

# Abbreviations

A. baumanni: Acinetobacter baumanni

A. hydrophila: Aeromonas hydrophila

AHA: American Heart Association

AIDS: Acquired immunodeficiency syndrome

ALT: Alanine aminotransferase

ASO: Antistreptolysin O

ATL: Adult T-cell leukemia/ lymphoma

B. burgdorferi: Borrelia burgdorferi

B. fragilis: Bacteroides fragilis

B. hominis: Blastocystis hominis

B. pertussis: Bordetella pertussis

B. (Rochalimaea) henselae: Bartonella (Rochalimaea) henselae

BCG: Bacille Calmette-Guérin

C. albicans: Candida albicans

C. canimorsus: Capnocytophaga canimorsus

C. difficile: Clostridium difficile

C. diphtheriae: Corynebacterium diphtheriae

C. haemolyticum: Corynebacterium haemolyticum

C. jejuni: Campylobacter jejuni

C. neoformans: Cryptococcus neoformans

C. perfringens: Clostridium perfringens

C. pneumoniae: Chlamydia pneumoniae

C. tetani: Clostridium tetani

C. torulopsis: Candida torulopsis

C. trachomatis: Chlamydia trachomatis

CDAD: Clostridium difficile–associated diarrhea

CFS: Chronic fatigue syndrome

CMV: Cytomegalovirus

CSF: Cerebrospinal fluid

CT: Computed tomography

DNA: Deoxyribonucleic acid

$D_5W$: 5% aqueous dextrose solution

E. corrodens: Eikenella corrodens

E. faecalis: Enterococcus faecalis

E. faecium: Enterococcus faecium

E. histolytica: Entamoeba histolytica

e. migrans: Erythema migrans

E. rhusiopathiae: Erysipelothrix rhusiopathiae

EBNA: Epstein-Barr nucleic acid

EBV: Epstein-Barr virus

EIA: Enzyme-linked immunoassay

ELISA: Enzyme-linked immunosorbent assay

ERCP: Endoscopic retrograde cholangiopancreatography

ESR: Erythrocyte sedimentation rate

F. tularensis: Francisella tularensis

FAMA: Fluorescence antibody to membrane antigen

FTA-ABS: Fluorescent treponemal antibody absorption

GBS: Guillain-Barré syndrome

GFR: Glomerular filtration rate
GGT: Gamma-glutamyltranspeptidase
*H. influenzae: Haemophilus influenzae*
HBcAb: Hepatitis B core antibody
HBsAb: Hepatitis B surface antibody
HBsAg: Hepatitis B surface antigen
HBV: Hepatitis B virus
HCV: Hepatitis C virus
Hib: *Haemophilus influenzae* type B
HICPAC: Hospital Infection Control Practices Advisory Committee
HIV: Human immunodeficiency virus
HLA: Human or histocompatibility leukocyte antigen
HPV-B19: Human parvovirus B19
HSV: Herpes simplex virus
HTLV-I: Human T-lymphotropic virus type I
HTLV-II: Human T-lymphotropic virus type II
ICU: Intensive care unit
IFA: Indirect fluorescence antibody
IG: Immunoglobulin
IM: Intramuscularly
IV: Intravenously
*L. pneumophila: Legionella pneumophila*
*L. reclusa: Loxosceles reclusa*
LA: Latex agglutination
LCM: Lymphocytic choriomeningitis
LDH: Lactic dehydrogenase
*M. avium: Mycobacterium avium*
*M. catarrhalis: Moraxella catarrhalis*
*M. fortuitum: Mycobacterium fortuitum*
*M. gordonae: Mycobacterium gordonae*
*M. kansasii: Mycobacterium kansasii*

*M. marinum: Mycobacterium marinum*
*M. pneumoniae: Mycoplasma pneumoniae*
*M. tuberculosis: Mycobacterium tuberculosis*
*M. xenopi: Mycobacterium xenopi*
MHA-TP: Microhemagglutination assay for *Treponema pallidum*
MMR: Measles-mumps-rubella
MRI: Magnetic resonance imaging
MRSA: Methicillin-resistant *Staphylococcus aureus*
*N. gonorrhoeae: Neisseria gonorrhoeae*
*N. meningitidis: Neisseria meningitidis*
OPV: Oral polio vaccine
*P. acnes: Propionibacterium acnes*
*P. aeruginosa: Pseudomonas aeruginosa*
*P. falciparum: Plasmodium falciparum*
*P. multocida: Pasteurella multocida*
PCR: Polymerase chain reaction
PMN: Polymorphonuclear neutrophil
PO: By mouth
PPD: Purified protein derivative
RIBA: Recombinant immunoblot assay
RMSF: Rocky Mountain spotted fever
RNA: Ribonucleic acid
RPR: Rapid plasma reagin
*S. aureus: Staphylococcus aureus*
*S. epidermidis: Staphylococcus epidermidis*
*S. equisimilis: Streptococcus equisimilis*
*S. minus: Spirillum minus*
*S. moniliformis: Streptobacillus moniliformis*

*S. pneumoniae: Streptococcus pneumoniae*
*S. pyogenes: Streptococcus pyogenes*
*S. saprophyticus: Staphylococcus saprophyticus*
SBP: Spontaneous bacterial peritonitis
SGOT: Serum glutamate oxaloacetate transaminase
SGPT: Serum glutamate pyruvate transaminase
SLE: Systemic lupus erythematosus

*T. glabrata: Torulopsis glabrata*
*T. pallidum: Treponema pallidum*
TA: Teichoic acid
UTI: Urinary tract infection
UVA: Ultraviolet A rays
*V. vulnificus: Vibrio vulnificus*
VCA: Viral capsid antigen
VDRL: Venereal disease research laboratory
VZIG: Varicella-zoster immune globulin
VZV: Varicella-zoster virus

# Acyclovir

 What dosages of acyclovir and duration of therapy are recommended for treatment of genital herpes simplex virus (HSV), herpes zoster, and varicella infections in patients with normal renal function?

## GENITAL HSV INFECTION

- Initial episode, normal host, and less severe cases:
  200 mg PO 5×/day for 10 days
- Initial episode, more severe cases:
  5 mg/kg IV every 8 hrs for 5 days
- Recurrent episode:
  200 mg PO 5×/day for 5 days
- Suppression:
  400 mg PO 2×/day. Dose may be titrated as needed. Treatment should be interrupted every 12 months to reassess the need for continued suppression.

## HERPES ZOSTER

- Normal host:
  800 mg PO 5×/day for 7 days to be initiated within 48 hrs of onset of rash
- Immunocompromised patient:
  10 mg/kg IV every 8 hrs for 7 to 10 days

## VARICELLA (CHICKEN POX)

- Normal host with normal renal function:
  Children: 20 mg/kg PO 4×/day for 5 days
  Adolescents/adults: 800 mg PO 4×/day for 5 days

Note: *Ideally, treatment should be initiated within 24 hrs of the onset of skin lesions.*

### SUGGESTED READINGS

Balfour HH Jr et al: Acyclovir treatment of varicella in otherwise healthy adolescents, *J Pediatr* 120:627-633, 1992.

Dunkle LM et al: A controlled trial of acyclovir for chickenpox in normal children, *N Engl J Med* 325:1539-1544, 1991.

Feder HM Jr: Treatment of adult chickenpox with oral acyclovir, *Arch Intern Med* 150:2061-2065, 1990.

Whitley RJ, Gnann JW Jr: Acyclovir: a decade later, *N Engl J Med* 327:782-789, 1992.

 Is use of acyclovir safe during pregnancy?

No increase in the risk to the mother or fetus has been documented with the use of acyclovir, but the total number of monitored pregnancies has been too small to detect potentially real but infrequent adverse reactions. The use of acyclovir seems to be particularly indicated in treatable conditions with potentially severe consequences during pregnancy (e.g., disseminated primary herpes simplex infections and maternal varicella pneumonia).

### SUGGESTED READINGS

Andrews EB et al: Acyclovir in pregnancy registry: six year's experience. The Acyclovir in Pregnancy Registry Advisory Committee, *Obstet Gynecol* 79:7-13, 1992.

Smego RA, Asperilla MO: Use of acyclovir for varicella pneumonia during pregnancy, *Obstet Gynecol* 78:1112-1116, 1991.
Spangler JG, Kirk JK, Knudson MP: Uses and safety of acyclovir in pregnancy, *Fam Pract* 38:186-191, 1994.

 Is acyclovir effective in preventing varicella?

Acyclovir (starting 7 to 9 days after exposure, 40 to 80 mg/kg daily in four divided doses for 5 to 7 days) appears to be effective in reducing the likelihood of developing clinical manifestation of varicella in infants and children following exposure in a household setting (16% vs. 68%) and in diminishing the severity of skin rashes. Of note, 76% to 84% of subjects receiving acyclovir have been observed to seroconvert, indicating subclinical infection in the majority of cases. Whether immunity derived from subclinical infection as a result of acyclovir treatment persists lifelong is not known at this time. At the present time, routine prophylaxis with acyclovir for prevention of varicella cannot be recommended. However, it may be considered as an alternative to varicella-zoster immunoglobulin and varicella vaccine, especially when these products are not available and it has been more than 4 days since varicella exposure has occurred.

## SUGGESTED READINGS

Asano Y et al: Postexposure prophylaxis of varicella in family contact by oral acyclovir, *Pediatrics* 92:219-222, 1993.
Huang YC, Lin TY, Chiu CH: Acyclovir prophylaxis of varicella after household exposure, *Pediatr Infect Dis* 14:152-154, 1995.

# Arthritis

 What are some infectious and noninfectious causes of "culture-negative" arthritis?

Several conditions may mimic septic arthritis, including rheumatoid arthritis, gout, pseudogout, Still's disease, Reiter's syndrome (urethritis and conjunctivitis may not be initially present), sarcoidosis, Sweet's syndrome, familial Mediterranean fever, Behçet's disease, acute rheumatic fever, and arthritis associated with inflammatory bowel disease. Infective endocarditis and Whipple's disease are often associated with "culture-negative" joint effusions. Occasionally, arthropathy may occur following rubella vaccination, particularly in women.

As much as 20% or more of septic arthritis cases may be culture negative, possibly related to factors such as the fastidious nature of some organisms for growth in the laboratory and prior antibiotic therapy. Organisms that may be more difficult to culture from synovial fluid or may require special media include mycobacteria, fungi, *Brucella* spp., *Borrelia burgdorferi* (agent of Lyme disease), *Neisseria gonorrhoeae, Neisseria meningitidis,* and viruses. The latter group of organisms includes hepatitis B, hepatitis C, parvovirus B19, rubella, mumps, lymphocytic choriomeningitis virus, HTLV-I, HIV-1, influenza, Epstein-Barr virus, adenovirus, and echovirus.

## SUGGESTED READINGS

Smith JW, Piercy EA: Infectious arthritis. In Mandell GL, Bennett JE, Dolin R, eds: *Principles and practices of infectious diseases,* ed 4, New York, 1995, Churchill Livingstone.

Studahl M et al: Septic arthritis of the knee: a 10 year review and long-term follow-up using a new scoring system, *Scand J Infect Dis* 26:85-93, 1994.

Totemchokchyakarn K, Ball GV: Arthritis of systemic disease, *Am J Med* 101:642-647, 1996.

Vincent GM, Amirault JD: Septic arthritis in the elderly, *Clin Orthop* 251:241-245, 1990.

How should bacterial arthritis be managed and treated?

Early diagnosis and treatment are essential to a favorable outcome in infected joints. Definitive diagnosis often requires arthrocentesis with appropriate cultures and gram stains. In nongonococcal arthritis, gram stain of the joint fluid is positive in 50% to 75% of cases, joint fluid cultures are positive in 85% to 95%, and blood cultures are positive in about 50%. In gonococcal arthritis, gram stain and culture of the joint fluid are positive in 25% or less of cases, and blood cultures are positive in only 10%; genitourinary cultures are positive in 80% of cases, however.

Treatment of arthritis caused by common bacterial isolates such as *Staphylococcus aureus,* aerobic gram-negative bacilli (e.g., *Escherichia coli),* and *Streptococcus* spp. requires removal or drainage of all infected joint effusion including inflammatory cells, enzymes, debris or foreign body, and antibiotic therapy. In gonococcal arthritis, use of effective antibiotics and needle aspiration are usually sufficient to eradicate joint infection. In patients with nongonococcal bacterial arthritis, surgical drainage (either open or by arthroscopy) with lavage is usually indicated.

For certain joints such as the knee, visualization of all compartments and efficient drainage and lavage are possible by arthroscopy without the attendant morbidity of open surgical procedure. Initial open drainage is advisable for infected hips.

Antibiotic therapy should be based on the in vitro susceptibility of the implicated pathogen. Although the optimal duration of antibiotic therapy is often unknown, most patients with nongonococcal bacterial arthritis are treated with 4 to 6 weeks of parenteral antibiotics.

Gonococcal arthritis should be treated with ceftriaxone 1 g IM or IV 1×/day, cefotaxime 1 g IV every 8 hrs, or ceftizoxime 1 g IV every 8 hrs; spectinomycin 2 g IM every 12 hrs should be used for ß-lactam–allergic patients. All regimens should be continued for 1 to 2 days after improvement begins, then switched to cefixime 400 mg PO 2×/day or ciprofloxacin 500 mg PO 2×/day (contraindicated in children, adolescents younger than 17 years of age, pregnancy, and lactating women) to complete at least a 7-day course.

Prosthetic joint infections often require removal of the prosthesis and intravenous antibiotic therapy. Occasionally, when detected early, some cases of prosthetic joint infection can be managed with open drainage, debridement, and antibiotics without joint removal.

Clinical observations have documented deleterious effects of prolonged immobilization on synovial joints, muscular atrophy, disuse osteoporosis, and late degenerative arthritis. In contrast, early active motion has been associated with beneficial effects on infected joints. Close follow-up of patients with septic arthritis for complications such as osteomyelitis, abscess formation, and progressive loss of joint motion is recommended.

## SUGGESTED READINGS

Centers for Disease Control and Prevention: 1993 sexually transmitted diseases treatment guidelines, *MMWR* 42(RR-14):61-62, 1993.

Esterhai JL Jr, Gelb I: Adult septic arthritis, *Orthop Clin North Am* 22:503-514, 1991.

Goldenberg DL, Reed JI: Bacterial arthritis, *N Engl J Med* 312:764-771, 1985.

Vincent GM, Amirault JD: Septic arthritis in the elderly, *Clin Orthop* 251:241-245, 1990.

# Asplenia

**Q** What preventive measures should be taken by those without a spleen to reduce their risk of severe infection?

## IMMUNIZATIONS

Vaccination against *Streptococcus pneumoniae* (at least 2 weeks before splenectomy, if possible, to ensure maximal antibody response) is strongly recommended for children 2 years of age and older as well as for adults with functional or anatomical asplenia. *Haemophilus influenzae* type b conjugate vaccine and quadrivalent meningococcal vaccine are also recommended, particularly in children. There are no known contraindications to administration of these vaccines at the same time, at different sites using separate syringes.

## PROPHYLACTIC ANTIBIOTICS

Chronic prophylactic antibiotic against pneumococcal infection is commonly recommended for asplenic children, irrespective of vaccination status. Commonly used regimens include oral penicillin V 125 mg 2×/day for children younger than 5 years and 250 mg 2×/day for those 5 years and older; amoxicillin 20 mg/kg/day may also be used for children younger than 5 years. For infants with sickle-cell disease, antimicrobial prophylaxis against invasive pneumococcal disease should be initiated before 4 months of age, preferably by 2 months of age. In children with sickle-cell anemia who receive regular medical attention without prior severe pneumococcal infection or a surgical splenectomy, prophylactic penicillin may be safely discontinued at approximately 5 years of age. Otherwise the age at which prophylaxis should be discontinued is unclear, and some experts continue prophylaxis throughout childhood and in adulthood, particularly in high-risk patients.

Routine use of long-term prophylactic antibiotics in asplenic adults is controversial given lack of appropriately designed studies. Given the lower risk of sepsis in adults, poor compliance with taking medications long term, and the potential for side effects and development of antibiotic resistance, routine chronic antibiotic prophylaxis of asplenic adults cannot be recommended at this time.

When long-term antibiotic prophylaxis is used, its limitations must still be stressed to patients or their parents because sepsis may still occur. Therefore antibiotic coverage at the first sign of fever is important. For patients who lack ready access to parenteral treatment, a supply of oral antibiotics active against major encapsulated organisms (e.g., amoxicillin/clavulanate, cefuroxime axetil, trimethoprim-sulfamethoxazole) may be immediately started until definitive care can be obtained. Regardless, such patients should have close follow-up and evaluation because fulminant sepsis may occur even following institution of therapeutic doses of antibiotics. Although no blanket recommendations can be made, ceftriaxone is a reasonable choice of parenteral antibiotic in asplenic patients with suspected bacterial infection.

## OTHERS

There are insufficient data to recommend routine antibiotic prophylaxis for asplenic patients undergoing dental procedures. Because of the possibility of rapidly fatal course, asplenic patients at risk of contracting malaria should pay special attention to standard precautions designed to reduce contraction of this disease. Avoidance of animal contact such as dog bites (risk of *Capnocytophaga canimorsus* sepsis) and tick bites (e.g., babesiosis from tick bites) has been suggested.

All patients without functional spleen should be educated about the risk of fulminant infection and advised to seek prompt medical care in case of febrile illness. Use of wallet cards or bracelets to alert emergency caregivers is encouraged.

SUGGESTED READINGS

ACP Task Force on Adult Immunization, Infectious Diseases Society of America: Immunizations for immunocompromised adults. Splenic disorders. In *Guide for adult immunization,* ed 3, Philadelphia, 1994, American College of Physicians.

American Academy of Pediatrics: Immunization in special clinical circumstances. In Peter G, ed: *1997 Red Book: report of the Committee on Infectious Diseases,* ed 24, Elk Grove Village, Ill, 1997, American Academy of Pediatrics.

American Academy of Pediatrics: Pneumococcal infections. In Peter G, ed: *1997 Red Book: report of the Committee on Infectious Diseases,* ed 24, Elk Grove Village, Ill, 1997, American Academy of Pediatrics.

Fedson DS, Musher DM: Pneumococcal vaccine. In Plotkin SA, Mortimer EA, eds: *Vaccines,* ed 2, Philadelphia, 1994, WB Saunders.

Styrt BA: Risks of infection and protective strategies for the asplenic patient, *Infect Dis Clin Pract* 5:94-100, 1996.

Q    When should patients without a functional spleen be revaccinated with pneumococcal vaccine?

Persons previously receiving 14-valent vaccine should be reimmunized with 23-valent vaccine (licensed in 1983). All children 10 years or younger with functional asplenia should be revaccinated 3 to 5 years after receiving the initial vaccine. Older children and adults should receive another dose of pneumococcal vaccine 5 to 6 years after the initial vaccination. Revaccination once only is recommended at this time.

### SUGGESTED READINGS

ACP Task Force on Adult Immunization, Infectious Diseases Society of America: Immunizations for immunocompromised adults. Splenic disorders. In *Guide for adult immunization,* ed 3, Philadelphia, 1994, American College of Physicians.

American Academy of Pediatrics: Pneumococcal infections. In Peter G, ed: *1997 Red Book: report of the Committee on Infectious Diseases,* ed 24, Elk Grove Village, Ill, 1997, American Academy of Pediatrics.

## STIMULATING QUESTION

Should a person with functional asplenia with unclear history of pneumococcal vaccination receive this vaccine? Are there any adverse reactions from revaccination if by chance he or she has been vaccinated in the past couple of years?

Minor side effects such as erythema, pain, and induration occur in as many as one half of the recipients of pneumococcal vaccine, but they are generally well tolerated and self-limited. Local Arthus-like phenomena have occasionally been reported after early second doses of 14-valent vaccine but are rare after revaccination with the currently available

23-valent vaccine. More severe systemic reactions such as rash or fever are also uncommon. For these reasons, and given the potential for fulminant pneumococcal infection in persons without functional spleen, pneumococcal vaccination should be administered when there is any doubt about prior vaccination (author's recommendation).

## SUGGESTED READING

Fedson DS, Musher DM: Pneumococcal vaccine. In Plotkin SA, Mortimer EA, eds: *Vaccines,* ed 2, Philadelphia, 1994, WB Saunders.

# Bacteremia

 How long should pneumococcal bacteremia complicating pneumonia be treated?

Bacteremia complicates the course of 15% to 25% of patients with pneumococcal pneumonia and is associated with an overall case-fatality of 18% to 61%. Infectious complications during *S. pneumoniae* bacteremia include meningitis, empyema, and septic arthritis. For these reasons, and because pneumococcal bacteremia often complicates severe pneumonia, duration of antibiotic treatment (e.g., penicillin G, ceftriaxone, or vancomycin, based on in vitro susceptibility testing) should probably be longer than that of uncomplicated pneumonia. A 10- to 14-day course of treatment, possibly longer if infectious complications arise, is reasonable.

## SUGGESTED READINGS

Esposito AL: Community-acquired bacteremic pneumococcal pneumonia. Effect of age on manifestations and outcome, *Arch Intern Med* 144:945-948, 1984.

Markowitz SM: Pneumococcal pneumonia. Recognizing and treating this persistent disease, *Postgrad Med* 88:33-42, 47, 1990.

Ruben FL, Norden CW, Korica Y: Pneumococcal bacteremia at a medical/surgical hospital for adults between 1975 and 1980, *Am J Med* 77:1091-1094, 1984.

How long should bacteremia caused by *S. aureus* be treated?

*S. aureus* bacteremia may be associated with metastatic foci of infection and endocarditis. The risk of these complications appears to vary depending on the patient and the setting in which they occur. In older hospitalized patients with recognizable primary site of infection (e.g., intravascular catheter) and underlying diseases, the risk of development of secondary foci of infection or endocarditis is 10% and 3%, respectively. In contrast, younger patients with community-acquired *S. aureus* bacteremia without identifiable site of primary infection are at high risk of developing metastatic infection and endocarditis (93% and 57%, respectively).

All *S. aureus* bacteremias, regardless of source, require a minimum of 2 weeks of effective parenteral antibiotics. In most instances, indwelling central catheters should be removed. A 2-week course of therapy is recommended when (1) bacteremia involves a host with no valvular heart lesions or "seedable" sites and with normal humoral and cellular immunity; (2) primary focus of infection is obvious and easily removed (e.g., intravascular catheter) or drained; (3) clinical and microbiological response (e.g., clearance of bacteremia) to therapy is rapid (less than 3 days) after intravascular catheter removal; (4) there is no evidence of metastatic infectious complications during the first 2 weeks of therapy; and (5) careful follow-up of the patient can be arranged after discontinuation of antibiotics. A negative teichoic-acid antibody titer after 2 weeks of therapy in a patient with a benign clinical course would also support the absence of metastatic foci (see section under "Serology").

When there are doubts about whether any of the conditions are met or a metastatic focus of infection is suspected (e.g., endocarditis and osteomyelitis), parenteral therapy for 4 to 6 weeks is recommended.

SUGGESTED READINGS

Iannini PB, Crossley K: Therapy of *Staphylococcus aureus* bacteremia associated with a removable focus of infection, *Ann Intern Med* 84:558-560, 1976.

Libman H, Arbeit RD: Complications associated with Staphylococcus bacteremia, *Arch Intern Med* 144:541-545, 1984.

Mortara LA, Bayer AS: *Staphylococcus aureus* bacteremia and endocarditis: new diagnostic and therapeutic concepts, *Infect Dis North Am* 7:53-68, 1993.

Sheagren JN: *Staphylococcus aureus;* the persistent pathogen (second of two parts), *N Engl J Med* 310:1437-1442, 1984.

Waldvogel FA: *Staphylococcus aureus* (including toxic shock syndrome). In Mandell GL, Bennett JE, Dolin R, eds: *Principles and practices of infectious diseases,* ed 4, New York, 1995, Churchill Livingstone.

 What is the proper management of coagulase-negative staphylococcal bacteremia associated with intravascular catheters?

Because the majority (50% to 80%) of coagulase-negative staphylococci are resistant to oxacillin and cephalosporins, intravenous vancomycin is the drug of choice. Catheter removal was once thought to be essential to successful treatment of coagulase-negative bacteremia. However, more recent data suggest that the majority (approximately 80%) of bacteremias caused by this organism can be cured without catheter removal. The optimal duration of therapy is usually 5 to 7 days in nonimmunocompromised cases in which clinical improvement is seen within 48 to 72 hrs; immunocompromised patients may require longer course.

SUGGESTED READINGS

Hampton AA, Sherertz RJ: Vascular-access infections in hospitalized patients, *Surg Clin North Am* 68:57-71, 1988.

Raad II, Bodey GP: Infectious complications of indwelling vascular catheters, *Clin Infect Dis* 15:197-208, 1992.

 What is the proper management of enterococcal bacteremia?

See section under *"Enterococcus."*

## STIMULATING QUESTION

Are ceftriaxone (Rocephin) and ticarcillin/clavulanate (Timentin) effective in the treatment of *S. aureus* bacteremia?

Ceftriaxone, a third-generation cephalosporin, has good in vitro activity against oxacillin-susceptible *S. aureus,* and even though it is highly protein bound (with less free drug available to tissues), it has been shown to be effective in the treatment of *S. aureus* bacteremia.

Ticarcillin/clavulanate is an extended-spectrum penicillin with good in vitro activity against *S. aureus.* It has also been shown to be clinically effective in the treatment of oxacillin-susceptible *S. aureus* bacteremia.

SUGGESTED READINGS

Diem E, Graninger W: Timentin in the treatment of invasive burn wound infection with sepsis, *J Antimicrob Chemother* 17(suppl C):123-126, 1986.

Jacobs RF, Elser JM: Timentin therapy for *Staphylococcus* infections in children: results of a multicenter trial, *Pediatr Infect Dis J* 8:441-444, 1989.

Palmer SM et al: Bactericidal killing activities of cefepime, ceftazidime, cefotaxime, and ceftriaxone against *Staphylococcus aureus* and beta-lactamase–producing strains of *Enterobacter aerogenes* and *Klebsiella pneumoniae* in an in vitro infection model, *Antimicrob Agents Chemother* 39:1764-1771, 1995.

Soriano E et al: Ceftriaxone monotherapy for severe bacteremic infections. Spanish Ceftriaxone Study Group, *Chemotherapy* 35(suppl 2):27-32, 1989.

## STIMULATING QUESTION

What antibiotic should be used for treatment of coagulase-negative staphylococcal bacteremia in a patient with documented vancomycin allergy?

Coagulase-negative staphylococci from nosocomial infections are usually resistant to multiple antibiotics, including oxacillin, erythromycin, clindamycin, chloramphenicol, and tetracyclines. As in the case of oxacillin-resistant *S. aureus* isolates, oxacillin-resistant coagulase-negative staphylococci should also be considered resistant to all ß-lactams, including cephalosporins.

Because of the rapid emergence of resistance of these organisms to ciprofloxacin, use of this antibiotic cannot be recommended. Rapid development of resistance of coagulase-negative staphylococci to rifampin also limits the usefulness of this antibiotic. Trimethoprim-sulfamethoxazole may be a useful alternative against strains with demonstrated in vitro susceptibility to this drug.

### SUGGESTED READING

Archer GL: *Staphylococcus epidermidis* and other coagulase-negative staphylococci. In Mandell GL, Bennett JE, Dolin R, eds: *Principles and practices of infectious diseases*, ed 4, New York, 1995, Churchill Livingstone.

# Bite Injuries

 How should a bite injury from a stray cat be managed?

The essential elements of the management of cat bites are as follows:

1. Wound care: copious irrigation; debridement as needed; suturing not recommended unless injury to the face, in which case delayed wound closure should be considered

2. Standard tetanus immunization as needed; give primary series and tetanus immunoglobulin if patient has never been immunized

3. Rabies prophylaxis as dictated by local health department and the ability to observe the cat: rabies hyperimmune globulin (RIG, 40 IU/kg or 18 IU/lb, half infiltrated around wound and half given IM) and rabies vaccine given at the time of the initial visit (day 0) followed by rabies vaccine administered also on days 3, 7, 14, and 28

4. Antibiotic prophylaxis, especially to cover *Pasteurella multocida, S. aureus, Streptococcus,* and anaerobes: amoxicillin/clavulanate (Augmentin), cefuroxime, and tetracycline (in penicillin-allergic patients who are not pregnant) for 3 to 5 days are reasonable choices

5. Elevation and immobilization

**18**

6. Close follow-up for early identification of complications (e.g., cellulitis and osteomyelitis)

7. Report incident to the health department

**SUGGESTED READINGS**

Griego RD et al: Dog, cat, and human bites: a review, *J Am Acad Dermatol* 33:1019-1029, 1995.
Weber DJ, Hansen AR: Infections resulting from animal bites, *Infect Dis Clin North Am* 5:663-680, 1991.
Wiley JF II: Mammalian bites: review of evaluation and management, *Clin Pediatr* 29:283-287, 1990.

How should a bite injury from a stray dog be managed?

1. Wound care: copious irrigation; debridement as needed; primary closure may be considered for wounds not at high risk for infection (e.g., not involving hands, treatment initiated within 24 hrs of injury, patient not immunosuppressed, and wound not involving deeper tissues)

2. Standard tetanus immunization as needed; give primary series and tetanus immunoglobulin if patient has never been immunized

3. Rabies prophylaxis as dictated by local health department and the ability to observe the dog: rabies hyperimmune globulin (RIG, 40 IU/kg or 18 IU/lb, half infiltrated around wound and half given IM) and rabies vaccine given at the time of the initial visit (day 0) followed by rabies vaccine administered also on days 3, 7, 14, and 28

4. Antibiotic prophylaxis is not as routinely recommended (in contrast to cat bites) except when involving the following situations:
- Presentation greater than 8 hrs after bite
- Moderate, severe, or deep puncture wounds
- Diabetes mellitus
- Asplenia
- Immunocompromised host
- Facial involvement
- Hand involvement
- Amoxicillin/clavulanate (Augmentin), cefuroxime, and tetracycline (in penicillin-allergic, nonpregnant patients) for 3 to 5 days are reasonable choices

5. Elevation and immobilization

6. Close follow-up for early identification of complications (e.g., cellulitis and osteomyelitis)

7. Report incident to the health department

SUGGESTED READINGS

Griego RD et al: Dog, cat, and human bites: a review, *J Am Acad Dermatol* 33:1019-1029, 1995.
Weber DJ, Hansen AR: Infections resulting from animal bites, *Infect Dis Clin North Am* 5:663-680, 1991.
Wiley JF II: Mammalian bites: review of evaluation and management, *Clin Pediatr* 29:283-287, 1990.

There is a patient in the office who appears to have cellulitis following a dog bite. How do I decide if hospitalization and IV antibiotics are indicated?

Most patients with clinically infected bites may be managed in the outpatient setting without the need for hospitalization. There are no clear-cut criteria for hospitalization, but in general the more complicated the nature of the injury and the more severe the cellulitis, the more likely that close in-house observation along with IV antibiotics will be necessary. Appropriate formal consultation with orthopedic, plastic surgery, or infectious diseases specialists is encouraged.

The indications for hospitalization include the following:
- Systemic signs and symptoms of infection such as fever, chills, and toxicity
- Severe cellulitis
- Deep tissue injury involving joints, nerves, bone, tendon, or central nervous system
- Peripheral vascular disease
- Immunosuppressed state (either by medication or disease)
- Diabetes mellitus
- Significant hand bites
- Head injuries
- Poor response of infection to oral antibiotics or outpatient therapy
- Suspected patient noncompliance with medications or wound care

### SUGGESTED READINGS

Goldstein EJ: Bite wounds and infection, *Clin Infect Dis* 14:633-640, 1992.
Griego RD et al: Dog, cat, and human bites: a review, *J Am Acad Dermatol* 33:1019-1029, 1995.

My patient was just bitten on the face by another patient on a psychiatric floor. What should I recommend? Is testing for hepatitis B and C and HIV necessary?

Besides local wound care, tetanus immunization, surgical intervention (as needed), and antibiotic prophylaxis are usually recommended (e.g., amoxicillin/clavulanate or doxycycline [contraindicated in children and pregnant women]).

Although rare, hepatitis B and C and HIV have been reported to be transmitted by human bites. Therefore it is reasonable to test the biter for the evidence of infection caused by these viruses. If the biter is found to be seropositive for or infected with any of these infectious agents, the injured person should undergo follow-up testing similar to the protocol used for exposure of health care workers to the blood of infected patients (see sections under "Human Immunodeficiency Virus" and "Needlestick/Blood and Body Fluid Exposure").

Other infectious agents that have been rarely transmitted by human bites include *Clostridium tetani,* herpes simplex virus, *Mycobacterium tuberculosis,* and *Treponema pallidum.*

SUGGESTED READINGS

Dusheiko GM, Smith M, Scheuer PJ: Hepatitis C virus transmitted by human bite [letter], *Lancet* 336:503-504, 1990.

Griego RD et al: Dog, cat, and human bites: a review, *J Am Acad Dermatol* 33:1019-1029, 1995.

Richman KM, Rickman LS: The potential for transmission of human immunodeficiency virus through human bites, *J Acquir Immune Defic Syndr* 6:402-406, 1993.

Stornello C: Transmission of hepatitis B via human bite, *Lancet* 338:1024-1025, 1991.

Vidmar L et al: Transmission of HIV-1 by human bite, *Lancet* 347:1762, 1996.

I have a patient who apparently was bitten by a brown recluse spider. What should I do?

Management of the bite of a brown recluse spider *(Loxosceles reclusa)* has been varied and is somewhat controversial. Most bites are not serious and resolve without complications; severe localized reactions may require surgical excision, however. *It is generally held that immediate surgical treatment of brown recluse bites results in more complications than initial medical treatment and therefore should not be performed.*

Conservative measures such as cleansing of the bite site, use of cold compresses, administering analgesics, and avoidance of strenuous exercise and local heat are usually advocated. Tetanus immunization status should be current. Prophylactic use of antibiotics (e.g., erythromycin) has not been studied in a randomized controlled trial but is often recommended. Use of corticosteroids has been suggested for systemic signs such as fever and malaise. Patients should be closely followed for signs of skin necrosis, which may develop after the bite and may eventually require surgical débridement.

SUGGESTED READINGS

Carbonaro PA, Janniger CK, Schwartz RA: Spider bite reactions, *Cutis* 56:256-259, 1996.
Rees R et al: The diagnosis and treatment of brown recluse spider bites, *Ann Emerg Med* 16:945-949, 1987.
Sendovski U et al: Brown spider bites, *J Fam Pract* 31:417-420, 1990.

Q  A patient reports being bitten or scratched by a wild squirrel. Should I worry about rabies or other infections?

Lagomorphs such as squirrels and rodents are considered to have a very low rate (0.1% to 0.01%) of rabies infection even in areas in which rabies is endemic in other terrestrial animals. In contrast to bites from other mammals such as bats, raccoons, skunks, and foxes, rabies prophylaxis is not routinely recommended following squirrel bites. Scratches from squirrels do not require rabies prophylaxis.

Tularemia and rat bite fever (caused by *Streptobacillus moniliformis* or *Spirillum minus)* have been reported following squirrel bites; however, currently there are no recommendations for routine antimicrobial prophylaxis against these organisms in this setting.

### SUGGESTED READINGS

Fishbein DB, Bernard KW: Rabies virus. In Mandell GL, Bennett JE, Dolin R, eds: *Principles and practices of infectious diseases,* ed 4, New York, 1995, Churchill Livingstone.
Goldstein EJ: Bite wounds and infection, *Clin Infect Dis* 14:633-640, 1992.
Magee JS et al: Tularemia transmitted by a squirrel bite, *Pediatr Infect Dis J* 8:123-125, 1989.

## STIMULATING QUESTION

Is antibiotic prophylaxis indicated following a rat bite?

Rat bites are rarely associated with infectious complications (2%). Although some have recommended routine antibiotic prophylaxis (penicillin V-K for 5 days), this recommendation has not been widely endorsed because of the low rate of disease transmission.

## SUGGESTED READINGS

Olivarius F: Rat bites, *Cutis* 53:302-303, 1994.
Ordog GJ, Balasubramanium S, Wasserberger J: Rat bites: fifty cases, *Ann Emerg Med* 14:126-130, 1985.
Weber DJ, Hansen AR: Infections resulting from animal bites, *Infect Dis Clin North Am* 5:663-680, 1991.

## STIMULATING QUESTION

A patient of mine was bitten by a pet monkey. What should I recommend?

Monkey bites may be more serious and more prone to infection that those of other exotic animals. Immediate, thorough, and vigorous cleaning of wounds with strong soap, iodine, or bleach solutions is recommended to decontaminate monkey bite wounds.

Besides the usual local wound management, appropriate tetanus immunization, and consideration of antibiotic prophylaxis, specific preventive measures geared toward herpes B virus (found in Old World monkeys, particularly in rhesus/macaques) are in order. This virus is usually associated with asymptomatic infection in the monkey but can be transmitted to humans by its bite, causing progressive and often fatal neurological disease such as myelitis and hemorrhagic encephalitis.

The wound should be immediately cultured for herpes B virus and the animal screened for infection caused by this virus (e.g., serological testing). Antiviral therapy with high-dose acyclovir or ganciclovir is often advised in the case of deep wounds or ones inflicted by symptomatic monkeys. Prompt acyclovir treatment has been associated with limiting the infection to the primary wound site in some cases. The patient should be instructed to report immediately any skin lesions or neurological symptoms (e.g., itching, pain, or numbness) near the bite site. Close follow-up is recommended. The assistance of the Centers for Disease Control and Prevention and expert medical consultants should be sought.

## SUGGESTED READINGS

Artenstein AW et al: Human infection with B virus following a needlestick injury, *Rev Infect Dis* 13:288-291, 1991.

Benenson AS: Meningoencephalitis due to cercopithecine herpesvirus 1, *Control of communicable diseases manual*, ed 6, Washington, DC, 1995, American Public Health Association.

Centers for Disease Control and Prevention: Guidelines for prevention of *Herpesvirus Simiae* (B virus) infection in monkey handlers, *MMWR* 36:680-682, 687-689, 1987.

Goldstein EJ: Bite wounds and infection, *Clin Infect Dis* 14:633-640, 1992.

Straus SE: Herpes B virus. In Mandell GL, Bennett JE, Dolin R, eds: *Principles and practices of infectious diseases*, ed 4, New York, 1995, Churchill Livingstone.

# Blood Cultures

 What are some important factors to consider when drawing blood cultures?

The site for venipuncture is important. Femoral sites or sites associated with active dermatological disease should be avoided because of their higher rate of contamination. Meticulous skin preparation is essential to decreasing the likelihood of obtaining contaminated blood cultures. The venipuncture site should be initially cleansed with 70% isopropyl or ethyl alcohol, followed by 1% to 2% tincture of iodine or 10% povidone-iodine solution applied centrically. The antiseptic should be allowed to dry completely before venipuncture. Double application of alcohol may be used in patients with iodine allergy. The venipuncture needle does not need to be changed before inoculation of the blood culture bottles. Whenever possible, blood cultures should not be obtained through intravascular catheters because of the increased potential for contamination.

SUGGESTED READING

Smith-Elekes S, Weinstein MP: Blood cultures, *Infect Dis Clin North Am* 7:221-234, 1993.

How many blood cultures are necessary to diagnose bacteremia?

Two sets of blood cultures (15 to 20 ml/set) have a reported sensitivity of 88% to 99.3%, and three sets of blood cultures have been reported to have a sensitivity of 99% for detecting nonendocarditis-related bacteremia. Therefore no more than two to three sets of blood cultures are usually necessary for evaluation of patients suspected of having bacteremia.

SUGGESTED READINGS

Washington JA II: Blood cultures: issues and controversies. Principles and techniques, *Mayo Clin Proc* 50:91-97, 1975.
Weinstein M et al: The clinical significance of positive blood cultures: a comprehensive analysis of 500 episodes of bacteremia and fungemia in adults. I. Laboratory and epidemiologic observations, *Rev Infect Dis* 5:35-53, 1983.

 How can one tell if a certain blood isolate is a true pathogen or contaminant?

When isolated in only one of several blood cultures obtained, isolates such as coagulase-negative staphylococci, *Bacillus* spp., *Corynebacterium* spp., and *Propionibacterium acnes* can be presumed to be contaminants. Delayed growth of the isolate may also suggest a contaminant.

Note: *In immunocompromised hosts or those with prosthetic devices, isolates often considered contaminants are likely to be pathogenic when grown from multiple blood cultures.*

SUGGESTED READINGS

MacGregor RR, Beaty HN: Evaluation of positive blood culture, *Arch Intern Med* 130:84-87, 1972.

Smith-Elekes S, Weinstein MP: Blood cultures, *Infect Dis Clin North Am* 7:221-234, 1993.

## STIMULATING QUESTION

Can *Clostridium perfringens* isolated from a blood culture possibly be a contaminant?

Yes! In one study, 50% of *C. perfringens* isolated from blood cultures were considered to be contaminants.

SUGGESTED READING

Weinstein M et al: The clinical significance of positive blood cultures: a comprehensive analysis of 500 episodes of bacteremia and fungemia in adults. I. Laboratory and epidemiologic observations, *Rev Infect Dis* 5:35-53, 1983.

# Bronchitis

**Q** How should acute bronchitis in otherwise healthy adults be managed?

Although the cause of acute bronchitis in most otherwise healthy adults is not usually clear, viral etiology is thought to account for the majority of cases. *Mycoplasma pneumoniae, Chlamydia pneumoniae* strain TWAR, and *Bordetella pertussis* are the only bacteria identified as contributing to the cause of acute bronchitis in otherwise healthy adults. Gram stain and standard bacterial cultures of sputum have not been helpful in identifying bacterial cases or predicting response to antibiotic therapy. Specifically, the etiological role of *S. pneumoniae* and *H. influenzae* isolated from expectorated sputum of patients with acute bronchitis is unclear because these bacteria are often isolated from the upper respiratory tract of normal persons. Given the predominance of viral bronchitis, it should not be surprising that the majority of studies have failed to demonstrate effectiveness of therapy with antibiotics when compared with placebo.

*Currently, routine antibiotic therapy of acute bronchitis in otherwise healthy adults is not recommended.* Increasing rate of antibiotic resistance among common respiratory pathogens such as *S. pneumoniae* and possibility of superinfection caused by antibiotic-resistant organisms should further discourage this practice. Instead, a trial of either oral or inhaled beta-2 adrenergic bronchodilators seems reasonable given the results of studies demonstrating superiority of these drugs to erythromycin. Additionally, symptomatic relief of cough with dextromethorphan or codeine may be indicated. Adequate hydration should be ensured to prevent drying of bronchial secretions. Smoking should be discontinued.

It has been recommended that when the incubation of acute bronchitis in a family appears to be short (a few days to less than 1 week), viral causes are more likely and antibiotic therapy should not be routinely prescribed. In contrast, when the incubation period seems to be a week or longer, treatment with an agent active against *M. pneumoniae* and *C. pneumoniae* strain TWAR, such as erythromycin or a tetracycline, may be reasonable even though no study has been done to demonstrate the effectiveness of antibiotic therapy against these organisms.

## SUGGESTED READINGS

Gonzales R, Sande M: What will it take to stop physicians from prescribing antibiotics in acute bronchitis? *Lancet* 345:665-666, 1995.

Gwaltney JM Jr: Acute bronchitis. In Mandell GL, Bennett JE, Dolin R, eds: *Principles and practices of infectious diseases,* ed 4, New York, 1995, Churchill Livingstone.

King DE et al: Effectiveness of erythromycin in the treatment of acute bronchitis, *J Fam Pract* 42:601-605, 1996.

MacKay DN: Treatment of acute bronchitis in adults without underlying lung disease, *J Gen Intern Med* 11:557-562, 1996.

Orr PH et al: Randomized placebo-controlled trials of antibiotics for acute bronchitis: a critical review of the literature, *J Fam Pract* 36:507-512, 1993.

 How should acute exacerbation of bronchitis in a patient with chronic bronchitis be managed?

When considering acute exacerbation of bronchitis from bacterial causes, the following facts should be kept in mind:

1. Viral causes are frequently responsible for acute bronchitis in patients with chronic bronchitis, accounting for 25% to 50% of such bouts.

2. Chronic colonization of the respiratory tract with unencapsulated strains of *H. influenzae,* pneumococci, and *Moraxella catarrhalis* occurs in at least one half of patients before the onset of acute illness, making it difficult to incriminate these bacteria as the specific cause of acute bronchitis.

3. Other organisms such as hemolytic streptococci, *S. aureus,* and enteric gram-negative bacilli are uncommon causes of acute bronchitis in patients with chronic bronchitis and may contaminate the sputum by colonizing the oropharynx.

4. *M. pneumoniae* may account for some cases of acute bronchitis.

5. It is often impossible to determine clinically or microbiologically whether an acute bronchitic infection has developed in patients with chronic bronchitis.

Management of such patients should include cessation of smoking and measures to improve sputum expectoration (e.g., postural drainage, use of bronchodilators and mucolytics, and hydration). The effectiveness of antibiotics in this setting remains controversial. A short course (7 to 10 days) of treatment (e.g., amoxicillin 500 mg 3×/day, trimethoprim-sulfamethoxazole 160 mg/800 mg 2×/day, amoxicillin/clavulanate 250 mg/125 mg 3×/day, or erythromycin 250 mg 4×/day) has been recommended by some authors; drugs such as azithromycin, clarithromycin, and cefuroxime axetil should be equally effective. Others have advised against the routine use of antibiotics unless the patient has coexisting cardiopulmonary disease and a history of three or more acute bronchitis bouts in the preceding year. The ultimate role of antibiotics in the treatment of acute bronchitis in this setting is unclear.

## SUGGESTED READINGS

Ball P et al: Acute infective exacerbations of chronic bronchitis, *Q J Med* 88:61-68, 1995.
Chodosh S: Treatment of acute exacerbations of chronic bronchitis. State of the art, *Am J Med* 91(suppl 6A):87S-92S, 1991.
Reynolds HY: Chronic bronchitis and acute infectious exacerbations. In Mandell GL, Bennett JE, Dolin R, eds: *Principles and practices of infectious diseases,* ed 4, New York, 1995, Churchill Livingstone.

# *Campylobacter*

 Should *Campylobacter*-associated diarrhea be treated and with what antibiotic?

*Campylobacter jejuni* enteritis is usually self-limiting; even without specific antimicrobial therapy most symptoms resolve within 1 week. Fluid replacement and correction of electrolyte imbalances may be all that is needed. Antimicrobial treatment reduces the duration of excretion of *Campylobacter* in the stool but may not shorten the course of enteritis when therapy is initiated several days after onset of illness.

The following patients may benefit from antimicrobial therapy:

1. Those with symptoms lasting longer than 1 week or worsening

2. Patients with high fevers

3. Those with bloody stools

4. Patients with more than eight stools per day

5. Immunocompromised patients, including those with HIV infection

6. Pregnant women (*C. jejuni* may have deleterious effects on the fetus)

Most isolates of *C. jejuni* are susceptible to macrolides (e.g., erythromycin), quinolones, and aminoglycosides. Up to 25% of strains may be resistant to tetracycline. Susceptibility to metronidazole, trimethoprim-sulfamethoxazole, and ampicillin is variable. *C. jejuni* is almost predictably resistant to cephalosporins, penicillin, vancomycin, and rifampin.

Erythromycin (250 mg PO 4×/day for 5 to 7 days) is the treatment of choice for most cases of *C. jejuni* enteritis. Azithromycin 500 mg PO 1×/day for 3 days has also been shown to be effective in decreasing the excretion of *Campylobacter* spp. and shortening the duration of illness. Clarithromycin (250 mg PO every 12 hrs for 5 days) and clindamycin (150 to 300 mg PO every 6 hrs for 5 days) may also be effective. Ciprofloxacin 500 mg 2×/day and ofloxacin 200 to 400 mg 2×/day, both for 5 days, may also be used in the absence of any contraindication to the use of these drugs. However, increasing resistance of *Campylobacter* to quinolones will limit their use for treatment of these infections.

Note: *1. Unlike* Salmonella *infections, treatment with antimicrobial agents does not prolong carriage of* C. jejuni.
*2. Use of antimotility agents may prolong duration of symptoms and has been associated with fatalities.*

## SUGGESTED READINGS

Allos BM, Blaser MJ: *Campylobacter jejuni* and the expanding spectrum of related infections, *Clin Infect Dis* 20:1092-1101, 1995.

Blaser MJ: *Campylobacter* and related species. In Mandell GL, Bennett JE, Dolin R, eds: *Principles and practices of infectious diseases,* ed 4, New York, 1995, Churchill Livingstone.

Kuschner RA et al: Use of azithromycin for the treatment of *Campylobacter* enteritis in travelers to Thailand, an area where ciprofloxacin resistance is prevalent, *Clin Infect Dis* 21:536-541, 1995.

## STIMULATING QUESTION

How common are postinfectious complications following *Campylobacter* enteritis?

Rheumatic symptoms have been reported in 20% of patients with *C. jejuni* enterocolitis and may occur up to several weeks following infection. Reactive arthritis associated with *Campylobacter* infection frequently involves patients who carry the human or histocompatibility leukocyte antigen (HLA)-B27 phenotype. This type of arthritis cannot be distinguished from other reactive arthritides associated with *Shigella, Salmonella,* or *Yersinia.* Its pathogenesis is unknown.

Guillain-Barré syndrome is an uncommon consequence of *C. jejuni* that usually develops 2 to 3 weeks after the diarrheal illness. From 10% to 40% of Guillain-Barré cases follow *C. jejuni* infections, in part related to the common occurrence of these infections. Pathogenesis of Guillain-Barré syndrome in this setting may be related to antibody cross-reactivity between structures such as lipopolysaccharides on the cell surface and glycolipids or myelin proteins.

*C. jejuni* enteritis is also a potential cause of acute motor axonal neuropathy in China and other developing countries. This condition is clinically indistinguishable from Guillain-Barré syndrome, but in contrast to the latter, it affects the peripheral-nerve axon and spares myelin.

Other less common postinfectious conditions associated with *Campylobacter* infections include hemolytic anemia, carditis, and encephalopathy.

## SUGGESTED READINGS

Allos BM, Blaser MJ: *Campylobacter jejuni* and the expanding spectrum of related infections, *Clin Infect Dis* 20:1092-1101, 1995.

Blaser MJ: *Campylobacter* and related species. In Mandell GL, Bennett JE, Dolin R, eds: *Principles and practices of infectious diseases,* ed 4, New York, 1995, Churchill Livingstone.

Bremell T, Bjelle A, Svedhem A: Rheumatic symptoms following an outbreak of *Campylobacter* enteritis: a five year follow up, *Ann Rheum Dis* 50:934-938, 1991.

# Candida

**Q** What are some risk factors for development of oral candidiasis/thrush in an adult?

Oral candidiasis is often associated with one or more predisposing factors such as HIV infection, corticosteroids (systemic or inhaled), leukemia and other malignancies, diabetes mellitus, antibiotic treatment (especially those active against gram-negative anaerobic bacteria), neutropenia (i.e., as a result of use of cytotoxic agents), dentures, salivary gland hypofunction, and psychotropic drugs (e.g., chlorpromazine).

**Note:** *1. Because of the presence of* Candida *spp. in the normal human mouth, the growth of this fungus from oral lesions is not, by itself, diagnostic of oral candidiasis.*
*2. Because the singular role of antibiotics or corticosteroids in causation of oral candidiasis is often difficult to assess (i.e., the relative contribution of the patient's underlying disease state is not usually known), all "healthy" patients who develop oral candidiasis while being treated with these drugs should still be considered for further evaluation such as HIV testing and blood glucose monitoring.*

### SUGGESTED READINGS

Allen CM: Animal modes of oral candidiasis, *Oral Surg Oral Med Oral Pathol* 78:216-221, 1994.
Greenspan D: Treatment of oral candidiasis in HIV infection, *Oral Surg Oral Med Oral Pathol* 78:211-215, 1994.
Odds FC: Candida *and candidosis,* ed 2, Philadelphia, 1988, Bailliere Tindal.

How should *Candida* spp. isolated from sputum of patients be managed?

Although *Candida* spp. are commonly isolated from sputum and bronchial specimens, particularly those from ill patients, they are rarely the cause of significant pulmonary disease.

*Isolation of* Candida *from sputum does not prove the presence of yeast in the lung because the source of yeast might be the oral cavity.* Diagnosis of *Candida* pneumonia is based on demonstration of fungal invasion of pulmonary tissue by lung biopsy; radiographic and culture findings are not helpful. Bronchial disease in the absence of concomitant pneumonia is extremely unusual. When *Candida* pneumonia does occur, it often afflicts those with underlying illness (e.g., leukemia) and it generally occurs in two forms: local or diffuse bronchopneumonia arising from endobronchial inoculation of the lung and hematogenous infection from a distant source.

Even though growth of *Candida* from sputum is usually not associated with candidal pneumonia, it should not necessarily be ignored. In the appropriate setting, *Candida* growth from sputum may suggest the etiology of stomatitis, laryngitis, or esophagitis, or it may indicate heavy gastrointestinal and respiratory tract colonization and potential risk of dissemination.

### SUGGESTED READINGS

Edwards JE: *Candida* species. In Mandell GL, Bennett JE, Dolin R, eds: *Principles and practices of infectious diseases,* ed 4, New York, 1995, Churchill Livingstone.

Masur H, Rosen PP, Armstrong D: Pulmonary disease caused by *Candida* species, *Am J Med* 63:914-925, 1977.

Odds FC: Candida *and candidosis,* ed 2, Philadelphia, 1988, Bailliere Tindal.

How should recurrent candidal vulvovaginitis be managed?

Before initiation of antifungal treatment, diagnosis must be confirmed by appropriate culture. Noninfectious conditions such as allergic and hypersensitivity vulvitis are often mistaken for candidal vulvovaginitis. Although the definition of recurrent candidal vulvovaginitis may vary in the literature, it generally involves women with a minimum of at least three to four clinically and mycologically proven cases of infection within 12 months.

Following the diagnosis of recurrent candidal vulvovaginitis, every effort should be made to eliminate potential predisposing factors such as antibiotics and birth control pills. It may also be reasonable to avoid occlusive nylon underwear (e.g., pantyhose) because of its potential exacerbating effect on vaginal *Candida* carriage. Unfortunately, however, the great majority of patients will not have any identifiable risk factor for development of candidal vulvovaginitis, and chronic suppressive antifungal therapy may be necessary in these patients.

Initial antimycotic therapy requires an induction course of oral or topical vaginal therapy (e.g., fluconazole 150 mg as a single dose, clotrimazole vaginal tablet [one] or cream at bedtime for 7 days, or terconazole vaginal suppository at bedtime for 3 days), followed by oral ketoconazole 100 mg daily, or once-weekly regimens of fluconazole 100 mg PO or clotrimazole (500 mg) suppository. It should be noted that regardless of the type of maintenance therapy, cessation of treatment may be associated with clinical relapse within a short time in half of the women.

When azole-resistant recurrent vaginal yeast infection is encountered (e.g., caused by *Torulopsis glabrata),* boric acid 600 mg vaginally once daily in a gelatin capsule for 10 to 14 days (or until cultures are negative), followed by a maintenance regimen of alternate-day and then twice-weekly therapy, should be considered.

Although sexual transmission of *Candida* has been occasionally reported, it is unlikely that this mode of transmission is an important factor in the majority of patients with recurrent vulvovaginitis. Studies of the value of antifungal treatment of male sex partners of women with vaginal candidiasis have not shown any significant benefit.

Note: *1. Until further studies are available, management of recurrent vulvovaginitis in HIV-infected women should be similar to that described previously.*
*2. Safety of systemic azoles such as fluconazole during pregnancy and breast feeding has not been established.*

## SUGGESTED READINGS

Anonymous: Oral fluconazole for vaginal candidiasis, *Med Lett Drugs Ther* 36:81-82, 1994.
Edwards JE: *Candida* species. In Mandell GL, Bennett JE, Dolin R, eds: *Principles and practices of infectious diseases,* ed 4, New York, 1995, Churchill Livingstone.
Odds FC: Candida *and candidosis,* ed 2, Philadelphia, 1988, Bailliere Tindal.
Sobel JD: Fluconazole maintenance therapy in recurrent vulvovaginal candidiasis, *J Gynecol Obstet* 37(suppl):17-24, 1992.
Sobel JD: Controversial aspects in the management of vulvovaginal candidiasis, *J Am Acad Dermatol* 31:S10-S13, 1994.

How should oral candidiasis be treated?

Several agents may be used to treat oral candidiasis, including the following:

1. Nystatin oral pastilles (contains sucrose) 200,000 U, 1 or 2 to be dissolved slowly in the mouth 4 to 5×/day

2. Nystatin oral suspension 100,000 U/ml (contains 50% sucrose) as mouth rinse, 5 ml 4 to 5×/day

3. Clotrimazole (Mycelex) 10-mg troche to be dissolved slowly in the mouth 5×/day

4. Ketoconazole (Nizoral) 200 mg, 1 to 2 tablets daily

5. Fluconazole (Diflucan) 100 mg, 1 tablet daily

6. Itraconazole (Sporanox) 100 mg, 2 tablets daily

7. IV amphotericin is reserved for recalcitrant cases

Note:   *1. Duration of therapy should be individualized, but 7 to 14 days is usually sufficient.*
*2. Ketoconazole and itraconazole absorption is decreased in persons with reduced gastric acidity, including those on antacids and H-2 blockers.*
*3. Potential for drug interaction between azoles and many other drugs is significant. For example, they interact with phenytoin, warfarin, cyclosporin, and rifampin. Ketoconazole and Sporanox may also interact with terfenadine (Seldane), astemizole (Hismanal), and cisapride. Refer to the respective drug package inserts for full prescribing information.*

*4. In HIV patients with oral candidiasis, initial treatment for at least 14 days is recommended. Cases of fluconazole-resistant oral candidiasis in patients with advanced HIV disease (CD4 <100) have been reported. In such cases, higher doses of fluconazole (200 to 600 mg/day), itraconazole (200 to 400 mg/day), ketoconazole (400 mg/day), oral amphotericin (1 ml 4×/day), or IV amphotericin may be considered.*

## SUGGESTED READINGS

Baily GG et al: Fluconazole-resistant candidosis in an HIV cohort, *AIDS* 8:787-792, 1994.

*Fungizone oral suspension,* Package insert, January 1996, Bristol-Myers Squibb.

Greenspan D: Treatment of oral candidiasis in HIV infection, *Oral Surg Oral Med Oral Pathol* 78:211-215, 1994.

Perry CM, Whittington R, McTavish D: Fluconazole; an update of its antimicrobial activity, pharmacokinetic properties, and therapeutic use in vaginal candidiasis, *Drugs* 49:984-1006, 1995.

Sanford JP, Gilbert DN, Sande MA: *Guide to antimicrobial therapy,* ed 26, Dallas, 1996, Antimicrobial Therapy.

 How should esophageal candidiasis be treated?

In less immunosuppressed patients with milder cases of esophageal candidiasis, clotrimazole troche 10 mg (one 5×/day) or nystatin liquid (10 to 30 ml) 4 to 5×/day swish and swallow may be effective. For severely immunosuppressed patients (e.g., those who have AIDS), Diflucan 100 to 200 mg daily is recommended as the initial treatment; ketoconazole is less effective in this setting. Itraconazole 50 to 200 mg daily may also be useful.

Patients who remain symptomatic despite therapy should have upper endoscopy to rule out other causes of esophagitis. For patients with documented refractory candidal esophagitis, amphotericin B IV (0.25 to 0.3 mg/kg/day) should be considered. All patients should be treated for a minimum of 14 days following resolution of symptoms.

## SUGGESTED READINGS

Haulk AA, Sugar AM: *Candida* esophagitis, *Adv Intern Med* 36:307-318, 1991.

Kwon-Chung KJ, Bennett JE: *Medical mycology*, Philadelphia, 1992, Lea & Febiger.

Laine L, Dretler RH, Conteas CN: Fluconazole compared with ketoconazole for the treatment of *Candida* esophagitis in AIDS: a randomized trial, *Ann Intern Med* 117:655-660, 1992.

 What is the clinical significance of *Candida* isolated from peritoneal cavity of surgical patients?

The presence of *Candida* in the peritoneal cavity is usually observed in the setting of gastrointestinal tract surgical opening or spontaneous perforation of a hollow viscus and may be associated with intraabdominal abscess or peritonitis in about 40% of patients. Mortality related to infections has been reported to be significantly higher among those with infection compared with those with peritoneal *Candida* growth without infection (42% vs. 3%). Mortality rate in patients treated for intraperitoneal *Candida* before a positive blood culture is lower than in those treated after blood cultures become positive (17% vs. 67%).

The management of *Candida* isolated from intraoperative peritoneal specimens has been controversial partly because of the apparently benign clinical course of some patients without specific antifungal therapy and probably also related to the potential toxicity of parenteral amphotericin B. Nevertheless, systemic antifungal therapy is recommended in patients with *Candida* growth from peritoneal cavity in the setting of acute pancreatitis, recurrent perforations, anastomotic leakages, postoperative peritonitis, "heavy" growth of *Candida* on initial specimen, increasing amount of *Candida* growth in serial specimens, positive blood culture(s), or critically ill surgical patients.

Amphotericin B IV at an average total dose of approximately 500 mg (minimum 200 mg) has been shown to be effective. The role of other less toxic antifungal agents such as fluconazole in this setting has not been delineated well. Superiority of amphotericin B and 5-flucytosine compared with fluconazole in the treatment of *Candida* peritonitis in patients in intensive care units has been reported. Patients with *Candida* infection should undergo ophthalmoscopic examination to rule out *Candida* retinitis.

## SUGGESTED READINGS

Abele-Horn M et al: A randomized study comparing fluconazole with amphotericin B/5-flucytosine for the treatment of systemic *Candida* infections in intensive care patients, *Infection* 24:426-432, 1996.

Alden SM, Frank E, Flancbaum L: Abdominal candidiasis in surgical patients, *Am Surg* 55:45-49, 1989.

Calandra T et al: Clinical significance of *Candida* isolated from peritoneum in surgical patients, *Lancet* 2:1437-1440, 1989.

Marsh PK et al: *Candida* infections in surgical patients, *Ann Surg* 198:42-47, 1983.

Rantala A, Niinikoski J, Lehtonen OP: Early *Candida* isolations in febrile patients after abdominal surgery, *Scand J Infect Dis* 25:479-485, 1993.

Solomkin JS et al: The role of *Candida* in intraperitoneal infections, *Surgery* 88:524-530, 1980.

How should *Candida* growth from an intravascular catheter tip be managed in the absence of positive blood cultures?

*Candida* may be isolated from intravascular catheter tips in the setting of invasive candidiasis or as an isolated finding in an asymptomatic patient. In the latter scenario, *Candida* growth may represent contamination during catheter removal or catheter colonization. Although there are potential risks for candidemia and metastatic infection in patients with catheter colonization, the actual risk of these complications after catheter removal is thought to be negligible. Consequently, the need for systemic antifungal therapy should be determined by the clinical status of the patient rather than catheter cultures alone.

Febrile patients who are colonized with yeasts in two or more additional noncontiguous sites and who have a positive intravascular catheter tip culture have a 25% chance for subsequent development of invasive candidiasis. Therefore these patients should probably be treated with antifungal agents. Although the optimal treatment of intravascular *Candida* catheter infection without candidemia is unknown, amphotericin B, generally considered the "gold standard" antifungal agent for treatment of serious *Candida* infections, should be considered. Alternatively, in patients without neutropenia or major immunodeficiency, fluconazole has recently been found to be an equally effective alternative in catheter-related candidemia (primarily caused by *Candida albicans* and not necessarily nonalbicans *Candida* spp.).

## SUGGESTED READINGS

Bach A: Relevance of culturing *Candida* species from intravascular catheters (letter and author's reply), *J Clin Microbiol* 33:3080, 1995.

Khatib R et al: Relevance of culturing *Candida* species from intravascular catheters, *J Clin Microbiol* 33:1635-1637, 1995.

Rex JH et al: A randomized trial comparing fluconazole with amphotericin B for the treatment of candidemia in patients without neutropenia, *N Engl J Med* 331:1325-1330, 1994.

# Cat-Scratch Lymphadenitis

 How can cat-scratch lymphadenitis be diagnosed?

Traditionally, the diagnosis of cat-scratch lymphadenitis has been based on the fulfillment of three of the four following criteria:

1. A history of animal (usually dog or cat) contact, with the presence of a scratch or a primary dermal or eye lesion

2. Aspiration of sterile pus from the node or culture and laboratory data that exclude other etiological possibilities

3. A positive cat-scratch skin test

4. A lymph node biopsy revealing characteristic histopathological findings (e.g., granulomas with necrosis or microabscesses)

However, the lack of commercial availability and standardization of cat-scratch skin test and the concern about potential transmission of HIV, blood-borne hepatitis viruses, and Creutzfeldt-Jakob disease through its use have made the inclusion of the skin test in the diagnostic criteria for cat-scratch lymphadenitis impractical and obsolete. The increasing availability of other diagnostic methods such as cultures and serology is likely to simplify the diagnosis of cat-scratch disease.

*Bartonella (Rochalimaea) henselae,* the principle agent of cat-scratch lymphadenitis, can be isolated from blood if lysis-centrifugation blood cultures are employed; usual culture methods will not usually detect *B. henselae* bacteremia. Growth of the organism from direct plating of tissue or aspirate is possible but difficult. Regardless of the source of specimen or culture method, the incubation period is often prolonged, ranging from 5 days to more than 30 days. Polymerase chain reaction (PCR) has been successfully applied to the detection of *B. henselae* in lymph node aspirates (sensitivity 96%).

Serological testing for antibodies against *B. henselae* has been shown to be useful in the diagnosis of cat-scratch lymphadenitis. An indirect fluorescence antibody (IFA) test shows high titers (64 or greater) in nearly 90% of patients with active disease, compared with 3% seroprevalence at these titers in healthy controls. A more sensitive (95%) and highly specific (nearly 100%) test by enzyme immunoassay (EIA) is now commercially available, which detects both IgG and IgM antibodies against *B. henselae;* the latter antibodies are often found simultaneously in patients with acute disease, but occasionally IgM may be present for 2 to 3 weeks before the detection of IgG. Other historical and clinical features that may help in the diagnosis of cat-scratch lymphadenitis include the following:

1. About 90% of patients have a history of exposure to cats

2. About 75% of patients have a history of cat scratch or bite

3. Inoculation site is evident in 59% to 93% of patients (average duration 7 days)

4. Fever is present in 32% to 60% of patients (average duration 6 days)

5.  Adenopathy alone is present in 52% of patients (average duration 3 months)

SUGGESTED READINGS

Adal KA, Cockerell CJ, Petri WA: Cat scratch disease, bacillary angiomatosis, and other infections due to *Rochalimaea, N Engl J Med* 330:1509-1515, 1994.
Barka NE et al: EIA for detection of Rochalimaea henselae–reactive IgG, IgM, and IgA antibodies in patients with suspected cat-scratch disease, *J Infect Dis* 167:1503-1504, 1993.
Fischer GW: Cat scratch disease. In Mandell GL, Bennett JE, Dolin R, eds: *Principles and practices of infectious diseases,* ed 4, New York, 1995, Churchill Livingstone.
Nadal D, Zbinden R: Serology to *Bartonella (Rochalimaea) henselae* may replace traditional diagnostic criteria for cat-scratch disease, *Eur J Pediatr* 154:906-908, 1995.
Regnery RL et al: Serological response to *"Rochalimaea henselae"* antigen in suspected cat-scratch disease, *Lancet* 339:1443-1445, 1992.
Slater LD, Welch DF: *Rochalimaea* species (recently renamed *Bartonella).* In Mandell GL, Bennett JE, Dolin R, eds: *Principles and practices of infectious diseases,* ed 4, New York, 1995, Churchill Livingstone.

 What is the recommended management of patients with cat-scratch lymphadenitis?

The optimal therapy for cat-scratch lymphadenitis is unknown because most patients recover without specific treatment. General supportive therapy with analgesics, avoidance of trauma to the enlarged lymph node, and bed rest when fever and systemic signs of toxicity are present have been advocated.

Large-needle aspiration of fluctuant lymph nodes (10% of cases) may be necessary to relieve pressure and pain. Incision and drainage of the involved lymph nodes are usually not recommended because of the possibility of chronic drainage and effectiveness of aspiration. Surgical removal of the inflamed lymph node is appropriate when the diagnosis is in doubt (e.g., malignancy is suspected).

Although several antibiotics have been reported to have good in vitro activity against *B. henselae,* controlled trials are needed to determine if such drugs hasten the resolution of lymphadenitis and what their ultimate impact will be on patient care. Antimicrobial agents with reported in vitro activity against *B. henselae* include erythromycin, tetracycline, amoxicillin, azithromycin, clarithromycin, rifampin, chloramphenicol, second- and third-generation cephalosporins, trimethoprim-sulfamethoxazole, and aminoglycosides. Quinolones have variable activity, and first-generation cephalosporins (e.g., cephalexin) have suboptimal activity against *B. henselae.* Therapeutic failures with ß-lactam antibiotics for susceptible isolates suggest the possibility of survival of the organism intracellularly or sequestration in tissue compartments into which ß-lactam antibiotics do not penetrate well. Thus treatment with antibiotics with good intracellular penetration may confer an advantage.

Use of antibiotics may be appropriate in patients with prolonged fever, systemic symptoms, or severe lymphadenitis. Based on their excellent in vitro activity and clinical efficacy in bacillary angiomatosus and *Bartonella* bacteremic syndrome, doxycycline (100 mg 2×/day) or erythromycin (500 mg 4×/day) should be considered. The optimal duration of therapy is unknown, although long duration of therapy (approximately 4 weeks) has been advocated by some authors because of the potential for recurrence. Routine use of steroids is not recommended at this time.

SUGGESTED READINGS

Adal KA, Cockerell CJ, Petri WA: Cat scratch disease, bacillary angiomatosis, and other infections due to *Rochalimaea, N Engl J Med* 330:1509-1515, 1994.

Carithers HA: Cat-scratch disease: an overview based on a study of 1,200 patients, *Am J Dis Child* 139:1124-1133, 1985.

Dolan MJ et al: Syndrome of *Rochalimaea henselae* adenitis suggesting cat scratch disease, *Ann Intern Med* 1189:331-336, 1993.

Fischer GW: Cat scratch disease. In Mandell GL, Bennett JE, Dolin R, eds: *Principles and practices of infectious diseases,* ed 4, New York, 1995, Churchill Livingstone.

Margileth AM: Antibiotic therapy for cat-scratch disease: clinical study of therapeutic outcome in 268 patients and a review of the literature, *Pediatr Infect Dis J* 11:474-478, 1992.

# Cellulitis

Q   What are some common and uncommon causes of cellulitis?

Group A *Streptococcus* and *S. aureus* are the most common causes of cellulitis. Previous trauma, laceration, puncture, or an underlying skin lesion such as ulcer or furuncle predisposes to the development of cellulitis.

Patients with *prior coronary artery bypass surgery,* saphenous vein resection, and tinea pedis may be particularly at risk for certain forms of cellulitis affecting the "donor" lower extremity(ies). A combination of compromised lymphatic drainage and venous insufficiency secondary to saphenous venectomy may contribute to lower leg edema and propensity to cellulitis attacks. Although the etiological agent is unknown in many cases, groups C, G, and B streptococci have been implicated.

Groups B and G streptococci have also been implicated in causing *recurrent cellulitis* in the setting of lower extremity lymphedema secondary to radical pelvic surgery, radiation therapy, or metastatic tumor involving the pelvic lymph nodes. Vulvar and inguinal areas and bilateral lower extremities are commonly involved.

*Decubitus ulcers,* particularly those in the proximity of the anus, may be associated with cellulitis caused by aerobic or facultative aerobic bacilli (e.g., *Pseudomonas aeruginosa, E.*

*coli,* and *Proteus* spp.), *S. aureus,* streptococci, and anaerobic organisms (e.g., *Bacteroides fragilis,* and *C. perfringens).*

*Diabetics* may suffer from two different types of cellulitis. Non–limb-threatening infections involve no ulcer or a superficial ulcer not extending to subcutaneous space, lack of systemic toxicity, relatively minimal cellulitis (extending less than 2 cm from portal of entry), and no significant ischemia. *S. aureus* and streptococci are the major pathogens in this setting, with facultative gram-negative bacilli and anaerobes uncommonly isolated. In contrast, the limb-threatening form is more extensive and is associated with deeper ulcers extending to subcutaneous space and significant ischemia. The cause is usually polymicrobial, including *S. aureus,* group B streptococci, *Enterococcus,* facultative gram-negative bacilli, anaerobic gram-positive cocci, and *Bacteroides* spp.

In patients with a history of *breast carcinoma,* axillary lymph node dissection, and associated lymphedema, cellulitis (at times recurrent) of the ipsilateral chest or arm may develop. The etiological agent is usually not determined, although non–group A streptococci (i.e., group C and G streptococci) have been implicated.

*Perianal* streptococcal infection caused by group A *Streptococcus* is a distinctive form of cellulitis found primarily in children.

*S. aureus* has also been implicated as the major cause of a less common form of cellulitis involving the scalp known as *dissecting cellulitis of the scalp* or *perifolliculitis capitis.* Its pathogenesis is thought to be related to follicular plugging, secondary infection, and deep-seated inflammation, similar to that found in hydradenitis suppurativa.

*Eikenella corrodens* cellulitis is often associated with *human bite wounds;* in such setting, this organism is often found concurrently with anaerobes commonly found in the human mouth.

*P. multocida* may cause cellulitis in the setting of *cat bite or scratches,* as well as bites by dogs, opossums, pigs, rabbits, rats, wolves, and roosters. Most cases develop within 24 hrs after initial injury.

*Erysipelothrix rhusiopathiae* causes an erysipeloid cellulitis primarily in persons *handling fish, shellfish, meat, poultry, and hides.*

"Seal finger" is also an erysipeloid cellulitis occurring in persons sustaining bites or trauma associated with *seals, walruses, and polar bears.* The etiological agent of this infection is unknown.

*Aeromonas hydrophila* is found in water (e.g., *lakes and rivers)* and soil. It causes acute cellulitis after exposure of nonintact skin to these environmental sources (e.g., during swimming). It may also cause infection following bites of aquatic animals such as pirahnas and alligators.

*Vibrio* spp. (e.g., *Vibrio vulnificus)* can cause severe cellulitis with bullous formation or necrotic ulcers following trauma sustained *in salt water or exposure to drippings from raw seafood.* Patients with alcoholic cirrhosis, hemochromatosis, and thalassemia are particularly prone to severe forms of this infection with associated bacteremia.

*C. canimorsus* (DF-2) may be associated with fulminant septicemia and cellulitis following *dog bites or scratches, cat bites or scratches, and contact with wild animals* (e.g., bears, coyotes, and tigers) or cuts received from working on a farm. About 80% of patients have had a predisposing condition such as splenectomy (most common), Hodgkin's disease, trauma, idiopathic thrombocytopenic purpura, chronic lung disease, corticosteroid therapy, and alcohol abuse.

Less common causes of cellulitis include *S. pneumoniae, H. influenzae* (particularly on the faces of children), aerobic gram-negative bacilli (e.g., *P. aeruginosa, E. coli, Serratia* spp., *Proteus* spp., and *Legionella* spp.), and *Cryptococcus neoformans*. Many of these infections are particularly found in immunocompromised patients.

Note:  *Aspiration of the leading edge of cellulitis may be helpful in diagnosing the infectious cause in no more than 30% of cases and should generally be reserved when unusual pathogens are suspected (e.g., in immunocompromised hosts), when fluctuance is detected, or when initial antimicrobial therapy is not effective.*

### SUGGESTED READINGS

Feingold DS, Hirschmann JV: Cellulitis. In Gorbach SL, Bartlett JG, Blacklow NR, eds: *Infectious diseases,* Philadelphia,1992, WB Saunders.

Goldstein EJ: Bite wounds and infection, *Clin Infect Dis* 14:633-640, 1992.

Moxon ER: *Haemophilus influenzae.* In Mandell GL, Bennett JE, Dolin R, eds: *Principles and practices of infectious diseases,* ed 4, New York, 1995, Churchill Livingstone.

Simon MS, Cody RL: Cellulitis after axillary lymph node dissection for carcinoma of the breast, *Am J Med* 93:543-548, 1992.

Swartz MN: Cellulitis and subcutaneous tissue infections. In Mandell GL, Bennett JE, Dolin R, eds: *Principles and practices of infectious diseases,* ed 4, New York, 1995, Churchill Livingstone.

Weber DJ, Hansen AR: Infections resulting from animal bites, *Infect Dis Clin North Am* 5:663-680, 1991.

Which antibiotics should be selected for treatment of cellulitis?

Treatment of cellulitis should be based on the setting in which it develops and the antibiotic susceptibility of suspected or documented etiological agent. For group A, B, C, or G *Streptococcus*, penicillin G or V, first-generation cephalosporins (e.g., cefazolin), erythromycin, clindamycin, or vancomycin is usually recommended. Note that erythromycin may have variable in vitro activity against group C *Streptococcus* and that this antibiotic and clindamycin may have poor in vitro activity against group G *Streptococcus* (see section under "Pharyngitis"). For most *S. aureus* isolates, a semisynthetic penicillin (e.g., nafcillin), first-generation cephalosporin, or vancomycin (in case of severe penicillin allergy) is usually effective; for methicillin-resistant *S. aureus,* vancomycin is the drug of choice.

Empiric therapy of cellulitis associated with open wounds in *diabetics* should include coverage for aerobic gram-negative bacilli, anaerobes, and gram-positive cocci. Potential choices of therapy include cefoxitin, cefotetan, ampicillin-sulbactam, piperacillin-tazobactam, ticarcillin/clavulanic acid, clindamycin and gentamicin or aztreonam, and clindamycin and a quinolone (e.g., ciprofloxacin).

When cellulitis occurs in the setting of *freshwater* injury, an antibiotic usually active against *A. hydrophila* such as gentamicin, a quinolone, trimethoprim-sulfamethoxazole, or a third-generation cephalosporin should be included in the empiric regimen (in addition to antistreptococcal and antistaphylococcal coverage).

*E. corrodens* cellulitis may be treated with penicillin, ampicillin, amoxicillin/clavulanic acid, second- or third-generation cephalosporin (e.g., cefoxitin, cefotetan, and cefotaxime), and tetracyclines. Quinolones have good in vitro activity against this organism, but clinical experience is limited. First-generation cephalosporins (e.g., cefazolin and cephalexin), semisynthetic penicillins (e.g., nafcillin and dicloxacillin), metronidazole, and clindamycin are usually *inactive* against *E. corrodens*.

*E. rhusiopathiae* cellulitis is treated with penicillin G, ampicillin, third-generation cephalosporin, or a quinolone.

For *V. vulnificus* cellulitis, a combination of doxycycline and ceftazidime, or chloramphenicol has been recommended.

*C. canimorsus* cellulitis should be treated with penicillin G. Ampicillin, clindamycin, erythromycin, tetracycline, many cephalosporins, ciprofloxacin, and chloramphenicol have also demonstrated in vitro activity.

For *P. multocida* cellulitis, penicillin G, ampicillin, amoxicillin/clavulanate, ticarcillin, piperacillin, second- or third-generation cephalosporins (e.g., cefoxitin, cefuroxime, and cefotaxime), tetracyclines, ciprofloxacin, and chloramphenicol should be considered. First-generation cephalosporins, semisynthetic penicillins (e.g., nafcillin), erythromycin, and clindamycin should not be used because of their suboptimal in vitro activity.

## SUGGESTED READINGS

Goldstein EJ: Bite wounds and infection, *Clin Infect Dis* 14:633-640, 1992.
Sanford JP, Gilbert DN, Sande MA: *Guide to antimicrobial therapy*, ed 26, Dallas, 1996, Antimicrobial Therapy.
Swartz MN: Cellulitis and subcutaneous tissue infections. In Mandell GL, Bennett JE, Dolin R, eds: *Principles and practices of infectious diseases*, ed 4, New York, 1995, Churchill Livingstone.
Weber DJ, Hansen AR: Infections resulting from animal bites, *Infect Dis Clin North Am* 5:663-680, 1991.

Q   How should patients with recurrent cellulitis in the setting of lymphedema be managed?

Because recurrent attacks of cellulitis may lead to aggravation of lymphedema, which in turn may predispose to future bouts of cellulitis, every effort should be made to prevent such infections.

Measures to reduce edema in the affected limb such as compression sleeves or stockings should be considered. Moreover, special effort should be made to prevent or treat minor cuts or breaks in the skin involving the susceptible limb (e.g., wearing gloves when gardening; wearing a thimble when sewing; using an electric razor for shaving; and avoiding dry skin, sunburn, and injections in the affected limb). Suppressive antibiotic therapy should also be considered in patients with frequent episodes of cellulitis despite such measures. Benzathine penicillin G (LA-Bicillin) 1.2 million U 1×/month, penicillin V 250 to 500 mg 2×/day, or erythromycin 250 mg 2×/day are reasonable choices.

## SUGGESTED READINGS

Bertelli G et al: Preventing cellulitis afer axillary lymph node dissection [letter], *Am J Med* 97:202-203, 1994.

Sanford JP, Gilbert DN, Sande MA: *Guide to antimicrobial therapy,* ed 26, Dallas, 1996, Antimicrobial Therapy.

Simon MS, Cody RL: Cellulitis after axillary lymph node dissection for carcinoma of the breast, *Am J Med* 93:543-548, 1992.

Swartz MN: Cellulitis and subcutaneous tissue infections. In Mandell GL, Bennett JE, Dolin R, eds: *Principles and practices of infectious diseases,* ed 4, New York, 1995, Churchill Livingstone.

## STIMULATING QUESTION

A man was bitten by a catfish 2 days previously while immersing his feet in lake water (apparently the fish were attracted to his feet and would nibble on his toes, whereupon he would flip the fish out of the water for consumption). He now suffers from cellulitis. What antibiotic(s) should be selected?

In addition to the common causes of cellulitis such as streptococci and *S. aureus,* aerobic gram-negative bacilli such as *E. coli, Klebsiella* spp., *P. aeruginosa,* and *A. hydrophila* should be considered. A combination of cefazolin and gentamicin or ciprofloxacin is reasonable.

Note: A. hydrophila *is resistant to ampicillin and ticarcillin, and it has unpredictable susceptibility to piperacillin, ticarcillin/clavulanate, and tetracyclines.*

SUGGESTED READING

McGowan JE, Steinberg JP: Other gram-negative bacilli. In Mandell GL, Bennett JE, Dolin R, eds: *Principles and practices of infectious diseases,* ed 4, New York, 1995, Churchill Livingstone.

## STIMULATING QUESTION

Is it safe to use corticosteroids to decrease inflammatory response in the setting of cellulitis?

There are no systematic studies available that address this question. However, the use of another class of antiinflammatory agents (nonsteroidals) has been associated with fulminant necrotizing fasciitis. Presumably, the depression of cellular inflammatory response by these agents may impair phagocytosis and hinder clearance of microorganisms in tissue. Therefore until further data become available, use of corticosteroids as adjunctive treatment of infectious cellulitis should be discouraged.

SUGGESTED READING

Rimailho A et al: Fulminant necrotizing fasciitis and nonsteroidal anti-inflammatory drugs, *J Infect Dis* 155:143-146, 1987.

# Ciprofloxacin

 What role does ciprofloxacin play in the treatment of respiratory tract infections?

Ciprofloxacin has excellent in vitro activity against many strains of gram-negative bacteria causing respiratory tract infection, including *H. influenzae, M. catarrhalis, Enterobacteriaceae* (e.g., *Enterobacter* sp., *E. coli, Klebsiella* sp.), and *P. aeruginosa.* Among gram-positive organisms, *S. aureus* may develop resistance, whereas *S. pneumoniae* and other streptococcal species may not be highly sensitive to this antibiotic. It has excellent in vitro activity against *Legionella* sp. and has been found to be clinically effective in the treatment of respiratory infections caused by this organism in a limited number of cases. Its activity against *Chlamydia* and *Mycoplasma* is moderate and good, respectively.

Clinical studies have generally shown a favorable response to ciprofloxacin in the setting of both community-acquired and nosocomial-acquired respiratory tract infections. The efficacy of ciprofloxacin in treating pneumococcal pneumonia has been questioned because of conflicting reports ranging from good to poor clinical response. Lower response rates and development of pseudomonal resistance have also been reported in association with ciprofloxacin therapy of gram-negative respiratory tract infections. Emergence of resistance to quinolones in *S. aureus* (both methicillin-resistant and sensitive strains) is not uncommon (see section under *"Staphylococcus aureus"*).

Although ciprofloxacin is useful in the treatment of a variety of bacterial respiratory tract infections, it clearly has the following significant limitations:

1. Largely because of the borderline activity of ciprofloxacin against *S. pneumoniae* and clinical failures, this drug should not be used as a first-line agent for treatment of community-acquired pneumonia or uncomplicated respiratory tract infections (e.g., bronchitis, pharyngitis, or sinusitis).

2. Ciprofloxacin should not be used as monotherapy for severe respiratory tract infections when the putative pathogen is *S. aureus, P. aeruginosa, K. pneumoniae, or Acinetobacter* sp. because of increasing reports of resistance of these organisms to quinolones.

3. Because of the generally poor in vitro activity of ciprofloxacin against anaerobes, this drug should *not* be used in patients with respiratory tract infections in which a significant anaerobic component is believed to be present (e.g., community-acquired aspiration pneumonia).

## SUGGESTED READINGS

Ball P: Emergent resistance to ciprofloxacin amongst *Pseudomonas aeruginosa* and *Staphylococcus aureus:* clinical significance and therapeutic approaches, *J Antimicrob Chemother* 26(suppl F):165-179, 1990.

Bassaris HP: Inpatient treatment of lower respiratory tract infections, *Infect Dis Clin Pract* 3(suppl 3):S145-S152, 1994.

Bergogne-Berezin E: Antibiotic therapy in inpatient respiratory tract infections: position of quinolones, *Infect Dis Clin Pract* 3(suppl 3):S153-S160, 1994.

Gordon JJ, Kauffman CA: Superinfection with *Streptococcus pneumoniae* during therapy with ciprofloxacin, *Am J Med* 89:383-384, 1990.

Peloquin CA et al: Evaluation of intravenous ciprofloxacin in patients with nosocomial lower respiratory tract infections: impact of plasma concentrations, organisms, minimum inhibitory concentration, and clinical condition on bacterial eradication, *Arch Intern Med* 149:2269-2273, 1989.

Phillips I, King A, Shannon K: In vitro properties of the quinolones. In Andriole VT, ed: *The quinolones,* San Diego, 1988, Academic Press.

What is the role of ciprofloxacin in treatment of urinary tract infections?

Ciprofloxacin has excellent in vitro and in vivo activity against a variety of aerobic gram-negative bacilli, the major cause of urinary tract infections (UTIs). Unfortunately, primarily because of the widespread use of fluoroquinolones in the recent years (ciprofloxacin is the most widely used antibiotic in the world), an increasing frequency of antimicrobial resistance to this class of antibiotics is being observed even among traditionally susceptible organisms such as *E. coli* and *K. pneumoniae*. In certain countries, over 40% of *E. coli* and *K. pneumoniae* isolates have become resistant to fluoroquinolones. Activity against *P. aeruginosa,* another common urinary isolate, has also diminished, with certain locales reporting greater than 50% fluoroquinolone resistance. *These data suggest that unless the current trend toward increasing fluoroquinolone resistance is reversed, the utility of ciprofloxacin in treatment of UTIs caused by aerobic gram-negative bacilli will diminish.*

Ciprofloxacin also has some inherent limitations in treatment of urinary tract isolates other than gram-negative bacilli (see section under "Urinary Tract Infections" ). It has been shown to be an effective and safe drug for the treatment of UTIs in renal transplant patients.

Ciprofloxacin achieves high drug concentrations in the prostatic fluid and tissue, with levels 1.5 to 14.2 times greater than serum levels. In acute prostatitis, penetration of antibiotics is facilitated by acute inflammatory process, and treatment of this condition is usually successful with a variety of antibiotics, including ciprofloxacin. In contrast, chronic prostatitis poses a special therapeutic problem because of the inability of most antibiotics in achieving therapeutic drug concentration in the prostate in the absence of acute inflammation. Studies of the use of ciprofloxacin (500 mg 2×/day for average duration of 4 weeks) in chronic prostatitis have reported success rates ranging from 65% to greater than 90%. Infections caused by gram-positive organisms, anaerobes, or chlamydia may not respond as well to ciprofloxacin treatment.

### SUGGESTED READINGS

Car JF, Goldstein FW: Trends in bacterial resistance to fluoroquinolones, *Clin Infect Dis* 24(suppl 1):S67-S73, 1997.

Childs SJ: Ciprofloxacin in treatment of chronic bacterial prostatitis, *Urology* 35 (suppl 1):15-18, 1990.

Grekas D et al: Treatment of urinary tract infections with ciprofloxacin after renal transplantation, *Int J Clin Pharmacol Ther Toxicol* 31:301-311, 1993.

Sant GR, Wainstein ML: Therapy of urinary tract infections in the elderly: role of fluoroquinolones, *Urology* 35(suppl 1):19-21, 1990.

Weidner W, Schiefer HG, Brahler E: Refractory chronic bacterial prostatitis: a re-evaluation of ciprofloxacin treatment after a median follow-up of 30 months, *J Urol* 146:350-352, 1991.

 What are some common and uncommon adverse reactions associated with the use of ciprofloxacin/ quinolones?

Adverse effects of fluoroquinolones can be categorized as follows:

1.   Gastrointestinal disorders (e.g., nausea, diarrhea, dyspepsia, abdominal pain, and anorexia) are the most common adverse effects of fluoroquinolones, affecting 4% to 20% of patients. *Clostridium difficile*–associated diarrhea has also been reported.

2. Central and peripheral nervous system reactions (e.g., dizziness, restlessness, confusion, depression, eosinophilic meningitis, anxiety, seizures, sleep disorders, manic reactions, paresthesias, headache, lethargy, and ataxia) have been reported in 0.9% to 4.7% of patients, with disorders of the central nervous system (CNS) accounting for over 40% of all adverse events associated with ofloxacin therapy. Convulsions are more likely to occur in the setting of prior epilepsy, preexisting brain lesions, or concomitant therapy with certain drugs such as theophylline.

3. Cutaneous reactions/hypersensitivity (e.g., rash and photosensitivity) have been reported in up to 2% of patients. Drug fever, vasculitis, Stevens-Johnson syndrome, toxic epidermal necrolysis, and anaphylaxis have all been reported.

4. Special senses effects (e.g., diplopia, changes in color perception, blurred vision, decreased visual acuity, eye pain, retroocular pain, tinnitus, and reversible high-frequency hearing loss) occur occasionally.

5. Cardiovascular effects such as hypotension, tachycardia, and syncope have been reported.

6. Renal/urogenital reactions (e.g., interstitial nephritis, occult hematuria, decreased renal function, and acute renal failure) have been reported in 0.5 to 4.5% of patients. The majority of patients with acute renal failure secondary to quinolone therapy have been older than 50 years old.

7. Hepatic dysfunction (often associated with elevations of serum glutamate oxaloacetate transaminase [SGOT], serum glutamate pyruvate transaminase [SGPT], gamma-glutamyltranspeptidase [GGT], lactic dehydrogenase [LDH], alkaline phosphatase, and serum bilirubin) and cholestatic jaundice have been reported. Fatal hepatic failure caused by ciprofloxacin is rare.

8. Hematological effects include leukopenia (in about 1% of patients), eosinophilia, anemia (at times hemolytic), and thrombocytopenia.

9. Rheumatologic adverse effects occur in about 0.5% to 2% of patients and include arthralgia, myalgia, arthritis, and vasculitis. A curious disorder, unilateral or bilateral Achilles tendinitis or rupture, may occur during ciprofloxacin (as well as several other quinolones) treatment. Although the pathogenesis of this complication is not well understood, it is hypothesized that DNA of mitochondria of eukaryotic cells is affected by gyrase inhibition of quinolones because of its structural similarity to that of bacterial DNA. A combination of low numbers of mitochondria and high tissue-drug concentration in tendons may result in reduced energy supply to the tissue and subsequently lead to degeneration of the tendon.

10. Myasthenic symptoms associated with muscular weakness have been reported. Therefore fluoroquinolones should be used with caution in patients with myasthenia gravis.

11. Pseudotumor cerebri (benign intracranial hypertension) has been reported with the use of ciprofloxacin and ofloxacin. The pathophysiological basis for this reaction is unclear.

## SUGGESTED READINGS

Asperilla MO, Smego RA Jr: Eosinophilic meningitis associated with ciprofloxacin, *Am J Med* 87:589-590, 1989.

Choe U, Rothschild BM, Laitman L: Ciprofloxacin-induced vasculitis [letter], *N Engl J Med* 320:257-258, 1989.

Christ W, Esch B: Adverse reactions to fluoroquinolones in adults and children, *Infect Dis Clin Pract* 3(suppl 3):S168-S176, 1994.

Rollof J, Vinge E: Neurologic adverse effects during concomitant treatment with ciprofloxacin, NSAIDS, and chloroquine: possible drug interaction, *Ann Pharmacother* 27:1058-1059, 1993.

Semel JD, Allen N: Seizures in patients simultaneously receiving theophylline and imipenem or ciprofloxacin or metronidazole, *South Med J* 84:465-468, 1991.

What is the role of ciprofloxacin in the treatment and prophylaxis of biliary tract infections?

Ciprofloxacin is excreted at high concentrations in the bile and has been used successfully in the treatment of acute cholecystitis and cholangitis, particularly those caused by *E. coli* and *K. pneumoniae*. Therapy is usually by IV route initially and switched to oral preparation once the patient is able to take oral medications and has had a favorable response. Because of the relatively poor activity of quinolones against anaerobes, monotherapy with ciprofloxacin cannot be advised when these organisms are likely to be playing a role in the patient's illness.

Oral ciprofloxacin administered before and after endoscopic retrograde cholangiopancreatography (ERCP) in patients with biliary obstruction or over 70 years of age has been found to be effective prophylaxis against ERCP-induced cholangitis and septicemia in high-risk patients.

### SUGGESTED READINGS

Karachalios GN et al: Biliary tract infections treated with ciprofloxacin, *Infection* 21:262-264, 1993.

Mehal WZ et al: Antibiotic prophylaxis for ERCP: a randomized clinical trial comparing ciprofloxacin and cefuroxime in 200 patients at high risk of cholangitis, *Eur J Gastroenterol Hepatol* 7:841-845, 1995.

Phillips I, King A, Shannon K: In vitro properties of the quinolones. In Andriole VT, ed: *The quinolones,* San Diego, 1988, Academic Press.

Is use of ciprofloxacin advised for treatment and prevention of traveler's diarrhea?

Oral ciprofloxacin 500 mg twice daily for 3 days has been shown to eliminate or reduce traveler's diarrhea (primarily caused by enterotoxigenic *E. coli)* in 90% of patients; concurrent use of loperamide (Imodium) may confer some benefit during the first 24 hours but not beyond.

Prophylactic antimicrobial agents (including ciprofloxacin) are not routinely recommended for prevention of traveler's diarrhea because of uncertain risk of widespread administration of antibiotics and their potential for causing adverse reactions in travelers (e.g., photosensitivity, antibiotic-associated colitis, allergy, and yeast vaginitis). Prophylactic ciprofloxacin (500 mg/day) may be reasonable in certain high-risk groups such as travelers with immunosuppression or immunodeficiency (see section under "Gastroenteritis").

SUGGESTED READINGS

Anonymous: Advice for travelers, *Med Lett Drugs Ther* 38:17-20, 1996.
Centers for Disease Control and Prevention, US Department of Health and Human Services: *Health information for international travel* 1996-1997, Washington, DC, December 1996, US Government Printing Office.
Taylor DN et al: Treatment of traveler's diarrhea: ciprofloxacin plus loperamide compared with ciprofloxacin alone; a placebo-controlled, randomized trial, *Ann Intern Med* 114:731-734, 1991.

Is the use of ciprofloxacin indicated in prophylaxis of wound infection following nail puncture of the foot through shoes?

An estimated 3% to 15% of nail puncture wounds of the foot become infected, resulting in cellulitis or localized deep-seated abscess, and 0.6% to 1.8% become complicated by osteochondritis with or without septic arthritis. *P. aeruginosa* is the major cause of these infections (greater than 90% of cases). Before the development of fluoroquinolones, prophylaxis against *P. aeruginosa* in this setting was not an issue because of the lack of availability of a well-absorbed antipseudomonal oral agent with good tissue or bone penetration. Although ciprofloxacin in conjunction with surgical débridement has been shown to be effective in the treatment of such infections (including those involving the bone), its role as a prophylactic antibiotic in this setting has not been systematically studied and cannot be recommended at this time.

SUGGESTED READING
Raz R, Miron D: Oral ciprofloxacin for treatment of infection following nail puncture wounds of the foot, *Clin Infect Dis* 21:194-195, 1995.

 Does ciprofloxacin interact with warfarin (Coumadin)? What other drugs does it interact with?

Ciprofloxacin (as well as several other quinolones) does indeed interact with warfarin, resulting in potentiation of anticoagulation and an attendant increase in the prothrombin time. The mechanism of this interaction is not clear but may be related to displacement of warfarin from albumin-binding sites.

Several other drugs may interact with ciprofloxacin. Because of its potent inhibition of the cytochrome P-450 isozymes, ciprofloxacin interferes with the metabolism of methylxanthines such as theophylline and caffeine, resulting in increased levels of the latter drugs. Seizures associated with concomitant use of theophyllines and ciprofloxacin have been reported.

Gastrointestinal absorption of ciprofloxacin is reduced by concomitant administration of didanosine (ddl); magnesium/aluminum-containing antacids; and calcium, zinc, and iron preparations. For this reason, ciprofloxacin should not be taken within 2 to 4 hours of most of these medications. In case of ddl, ciprofloxacin should be taken at least 2 hours before or 6 hours after its administration.

Probenecid increases the plasma area under the concentration-time curve and elimination half-life of ciprofloxacin.

Concomitant administration of ciprofloxacin with glyburide may result in exaggerated hypoglycemic effect of the latter.

There are conflicting reports as to the degree of interaction between ciprofloxacin and cyclosporin. Nevertheless, it may be prudent to closely monitor cyclosporin levels when these two drugs are taken concurrently.

## SUGGESTED READINGS

Adam D, von Rosenstiel N: Adverse reactions to quinolones, potential toxicities, drug interactions, and metabolic effects, *Infect Dis Clin Pract* 3(suppl 3):S177-S184, 1994.

Jaehde U et al: Effect of probenecid on the distribution and elimination of ciprofloxacin in humans, *Clin Pharmacol Ther* 58:532-541, 1995.

Mott FE, Murphy S, Hunt V: Ciprofloxacin and warfarin, *Ann Intern Med* 111:542-543, 1989.

Polk RE: Drug interactions with fluoroquinolone antibiotics and patient education, *Infect Dis Clin Pract* 3(suppl 3):S177-S184, 1994.

Sahai J et al: Cations in the didanosine tablet reduce ciprofloxacin bioavailability, *Clin Parmacol Ther* 53:292-297, 1993.

What is the role of ciprofloxacin in the treatment of cellulitis and soft tissue infections?

Ciprofloxacin (as well as other fluoroquinolones) should not be used as a first-line agent in the treatment of most soft tissue infections because of their inferior activity against many gram-positive bacteria (e.g., streptococci) and variable activity against *S. aureus*. It may be a reasonable antibiotic choice when aerobic gram-negative bacilli are thought to be a cause of cellulitis (e.g., in the setting of diabetic foot infections or when *Aeromonas* sp. is in the differential). Because of its poor to marginal activity against anaerobes, this drug should not be used as monotherapy when a mixed infection involving anaerobic bacteria is likely.

SUGGESTED READING

Rubinstein E, Keller N: Fluoroquinolones: present uses, *Infect Dis Clin Pract* 3(suppl 3):S195-S202, 1994.

Under what circumstances should the use of IV ciprofloxacin be considered?

The daily cost of treatment with IV ciprofloxacin (400 mg every 12 hrs) is about 10 times higher than the oral form of this drug (500 mg 2×/day). However, serum and tissue concentrations are comparable between these two preparations, with oral ciprofloxacin usually having greater than 70% bioavailability.

Because of these reasons and because of increasing bacterial resistance, IV ciprofloxacin should be considered an alternative for the treatment of infections of the urinary and lower respiratory tracts only when the following conditions exist: (1) documented bacterial resistance to less costly agents; (2) documented hypersensitivity to first-line agents; and (3) inability to take oral ciprofloxacin because of inability to ingest or absorb.

### SUGGESTED READINGS

Anonymous: Intravenous ciprofloxacin, *Med Lett Drugs Ther* 33:75-76, 1991.
Anonymous: Intravenous ciprofloxacin: a position statement by the Society of Infectious Diseases Pharmacists, *Ann Pharmacother* 27:362-364, 1993.
Frisolone J, Manzo J, Leviton IM: Criteria for use of intravenous ciprofloxacin for infections in adult patients, *Clin Pharm* 12:226-232, 1993.
Lettieri JT et al: Pharmacokinetic profiles of ciprofloxacin after single intravenous and oral doses, *Antimicrob Agents Chemother* 36:993-996, 1992.

 Should the dose of ciprofloxacin be reduced in renal insufficiency?

Ciprofloxacin is cleared by both renal and hepatic routes. Its half-life is only modestly increased even in anuric patients, and its bioavailability is not affected by renal insufficiency. No reduction in dosage is recommended unless the glomerular filtration rate drops below 20 ml/min, in which case the daily dose is reduced by one half (usually from 2×/day to same dose 1×/day).

Note: *Not all fluoroquinolones have the same degree of renal clearance. For example, ofloxacin is cleared much more by the kidneys than ciprofloxacin, and it requires major dose reductions in renal insufficiency.*

## SUGGESTED READINGS

Bergan T: Pharmacokinetics of fluorinated quinolones. In Andriole VT, ed: *The quinolones,* San Diego, 1988, Academic Press.

Plaisance KI et al: Effect of renal function on the bioavailability of ciprofloxacin, *Antimicrob Agents Chemother* 34:1031-1034, 1990.

Scully BE: Pharmacology of the fluoroquinolones, *Urology* 35(suppl 1):8-10, 1990.

# Clostridium difficile–Associated Diarrhea

Q What is the best way to diagnose *C. difficile*–associated diarrhea (CDAD)?

Optimal criteria for diagnosis of CDAD include clinical evidence of diarrhea and either (1) evidence in stool of the organism, its toxin, or both; or (2) visual documentation of pseudomembranous colitis in patients with culture-positive stools only; in vitro demonstration of toxin production by the organisms should be confirmed.

The "gold standard" laboratory test for detection of *C. difficile* toxin in the stool has been the cytotoxic assay. This test is greater than or equal to 95% specific with a sensitivity of 67% to 100% for CDAD. Culture for *C. difficile* has a high sensitivity (greater than or equal to 95%) but a relatively poor specificity for CDAD. Immunoassay tests for *C. difficile* toxin generally have good specificity but lower sensitivity compared with the cytotoxic tests.

## SUGGESTED READINGS

Gerding DN: Diagnosis of *Clostridium difficile*–associated disease: patient selection and test perfection, *Am J Med* 100:485-486, 1996.

Gerding DN, Brazier JS: Optimal methods for identifying *Clostridium difficile* infections, *Clin Infect Dis* 16(suppl 4):S439-S442, 1993.

Peterson LR, Kelly PJ: The role of the clinical microbiology laboratory in the management of *Clostridium difficile*–associated diarrhea, *Infect Dis Clin North Am* 7:277-293, 1993.

Q    What is the best treatment for CDAD and its relapse?

The "gold standard" therapy has been PO (not IV) vancomycin (125 to 500 mg 4×/day). For mild to moderate cases metronidazole (250 to 500 mg 4×/day) is preferred because of significantly lower cost of the drug and the recent concern over emergence of vancomycin resistance in gram-positive bacteria such as enterococci. Relapse may be treated with oral vancomycin or metronidazole for 7 to 14 days. Anecdotally, those with more than one recurrence may respond to longer courses (4 to 6 weeks) of therapy followed by a gradual tapering of the dose.

Note: *Antiperistaltic agents should be avoided in patients with CDAD because of concern over promotion of injury to the colonic mucosa caused by toxin retention.*

SUGGESTED READINGS
Cherry RD et al: Metronidazole: an alternative therapy for antibiotic-associated colitis, *Gastroenterology* 82:849-851, 1982.
Fekety R: Antibiotic-associated colitis. In Mandell GL, Bennett JE, Dolin R, eds: *Principles and practices of infectious diseases,* ed 4, New York, 1995, Churchill Livingstone.

## STIMULATING QUESTION

How do you treat patients with CDAD who are allergic to metronidazole and cannot afford oral vancomycin?

Vancomycin elixir can be compounded from IV solution, which is much cheaper (but also less palatable). The dose is 125 mg orally 4×/day for 10 days.

SUGGESTED READING
Drapkin MS: Nosocomial infection with *C. difficile, Infect Dis Clin Pract* 1:138-142, 1992.

# Cytomegalovirus

 How should cytomegalovirus (CMV)-specific IgG and IgM antibody tests be interpreted?

CMV-specific IgG antibody may be present in both acute and distant infection. Testing for CMV-specific IgG may be useful in the following situations: (1) to determine suscepti-bility to primary infection (e.g., in women of fertile age or transplant recipients) and (2) to select CMV-seronegative blood donors who would be much less likely to transmit CMV infection to high-risk groups (2.6% vs. 16% to 30% for seropositive blood donors).

CMV-specific IgM antibody may be helpful in diagnosing acute or recent active infection. It may be elevated not only in primary but also in reactivation CMV infection. It is usually present in immunocompetent patients suspected of having acute primary CMV infection particularly from a week or more after the onset of illness and may persist for 6 to 9 months after the illness; thus its absence in this patient population during acute primary infection would be highly unusual. False-positive CMV IgM may occur because of persistence of antibody for several months following primary infection, in rheumatoid arthritis, in Epstein-Barr infections, and others (e.g., asymptomatic homosexual men). In AIDS patients CMV-specific antibody is frequently present even when clinically important infection is absent. For these reasons, CMV-specific IgM antibody test results should only be interpreted in the clinical context in which they are being ordered.

In certain severely immunocompromised patients (e.g., transplant patients), the ability to mount an IgM response may be impaired because of the underlying disease or immunosuppressants. Thus absence of IgM-specific CMV antibody in these patients does not rule out the possibility of acute or reactivation CMV infection.

When congenital CMV infection is being considered, absence of CMV-specific IgG in the infant essentially rules out this infection because seronegative mothers will not pass infections to their babies. Testing for CMV-specific IgM in infants in this setting is neither sensitive (33% by ELISA) nor specific.

### SUGGESTED READINGS

Cohen JI, Corey GR: Cytomegalovirus infection in the normal host, *Medicine* 64:100-112, 1985.

Drew WL: Diagnosis of cytomegalovirus infection, *Rev Infect Dis* 10(suppl 3):S468-S476, 1988.

Landini MP, Mach M: Searching for antibodies specific for human cytomegalovirus: is it diagnostically useful? When and how, *Scand J Infect Dis* 99(suppl):18-23, 1995.

Mangano WE, Gruninger RP: Use of viral cultures and serologic tests for cytomegalovirus infection. Rational or random? *Am J Clin Pathol* 106:180-184, 1996.

 How is CMV transmitted?

CMV transmission from person to person may occur in several different ways, including the following:

1. Heterosexual contact; semen and uterine cervix are thought to be important reservoirs of CMV in this setting. Condoms may help prevent sexual transmission of CMV.

2. Homosexual contact; receptive anal intercourse is highly correlated with acquisition of CMV infection in this setting. Condoms may help prevent sexual transmission of CMV.

3. Transplacental transmission; babies born to mothers who acquired primary CMV infection during pregnancy are at risk of developing symptomatic disease (19%).

4. Perinatal; via breast milk (accounts for up to 50% of transmitted infections from mother to infant) or during passage through the birth canal and exposure to cervical and vaginal secretions.

5. Organ transplantation (seropositive donor to susceptible seronegative recipient).

6. Blood transfusion; estimates of risk of transmission per unit of blood vary from less than 0.4% to 12%. HLA matching may favor transmission by increasing the likelihood of survival of latently infected donor leukocytes.

7. Day care setting; transmission may occur among children or from child to caretaker.

8. Household setting.

Additional considerations include the following:

1. CMV transmission from patients to hospital personnel occurs rarely, if at all, and has never been documented.

2. Patient-to-patient transmission of CMV is also considered to occur rarely and has been reported only in children under crowded conditions (e.g., neonatal intensive care units).

3. Environmental surfaces are not considered an important source of CMV infection; viral half-life is 2 to 6 hours on such surfaces.

4. CMV infection in immunocompetent persons is generally not associated with disease (i.e., it is usually asymptomatic).

SUGGESTED READINGS

Adler SP: Cytomegalovirus. In Mandell GL, Bennett JE, Dolin R, eds: *Principles and practices of infectious diseases*, ed 4, New York, 1995, Churchill Livingstone.
Ho M: Epidemiology of cytomegalovirus infections, *Rev Infect Dis* 12(suppl 7):S701-S710, 1990.
Katznelson S, Drew WL, Mintz L: Efficacy of the condom as a barrier to the transmission of cytomegalovirus, *J Infect Dis* 150:155-157, 1984.
Sayers MH et al: Reducing the risk for transfusion-transmitted cytomegalovirus infection, *Ann Intern Med* 116:55-62, 1992.
Spector SA: Transmission of cytomegalovirus among infants in hospital documented by restriction-endonuclease-digestion analyses, *Lancet* 1:378-380, 1983.

 In what body fluids is CMV found?

CMV may be found in blood (particularly white blood cells), urine, oral secretions, cervical secretions, semen, breast milk, feces, and tears. CMV is not usually detectable in the body fluids of normal adults except in their cervical secretions or semen. However, persons who are recovering from acute infection may carry the virus in the urine, throat, and occasionally blood for months. Others with congenital or perinatal infection or immunodeficiency, such as transplant patients, and those with AIDS are often chronic virus carriers for years.

## SUGGESTED READINGS

Ho M: Cytomegalovirus. In Mandell GL, Bennett JE, Dolin R, eds: *Principles and practices of infectious diseases,* ed 4, New York, 1995, Churchill Livingstone.
Naraqi S: Cytomegalovirus. In Belche RB, ed: *Textbook of human virology,* Littleton, Ma, 1984, PSG.

 What advice should be given to a pregnant health care worker who cared for a patient subsequently found to have CMV infection?

Early studies initially suggested that health care workers had elevated risk of CMV infection similar to that of day care workers. However, subsequent reports have not shown an increased risk, possibly related to the practice of universal precautions. Moreover, no increase in CMV infection among dialysis workers or renal transplantation workers has been observed. There has been no documentation of occupationally acquired CMV infection in the health care setting. For these reasons, health care workers (pregnant or not) who adhere to universal blood and body fluids precautions should not be considered to be at increased risk of CMV transmission from occupational sources and should not require special management as a result of their caring for a CMV-infected patient.

## SUGGESTED READINGS

Brady MT: Cytomegalovirus infections: occupational risk for health professionals, *Am J Infect Control* 14:197-203, 1989.
Dworsky ME et al: Occupational risk for primary cytomegalovirus infection among pediatric health-care workers, *N Engl J Med* 309:950-953, 1983.
Hokeberg I et al: No evidence of hospital-acquired cytomegalovirus infection in a pregnant pediatric nurse using restriction endonuclease analysis, *Pediatr Infect Dis* 7:812-814, 1988.
Sepkowitz KA: Occupationally acquired infections in health care workers. II, *Ann Intern Med* 125:917-928, 1996.

How should CMV isolated from blood or urine be interpreted?

CMV is not usually cultured from blood or urine of normal healthy adults unless they are recovering from acute CMV infection, in which case it may be found in the urine, throat, and occasionally blood for many months. Immunosuppressed patients such as transplant recipients and those with AIDS may have CMV in the urine or blood for years without necessarily having symptomatic disease.

CMV viremia correlates poorly with the presence of either fever or weight loss in patients with AIDS (CD4 <200). Lack of CMV growth from blood cultures of AIDS patients does not exclude CMV disease (sensitivity 55%). Viruria in this patient population is sensitive for CMV disease (88%) but has poor specificity and is not predictive of viremia.

### SUGGESTED READINGS

Ho M: Cytomegalovirus. In Mandell GL, Bennett JE, Dolin R, eds: *Principles and practices of infectious diseases,* ed 4, New York, 1995, Churchill Livingstone.

Zurlo JJ et al: Lack of clinical utility of cytomegalovirus blood and urine cultures in patients with HIV infection, *Ann Intern Med* 118:12-17, 1993.

 How should a positive CMV culture from bronchoalveolar lavage be interpreted?

CMV is usually not isolated from normal adults, except during acute infection. In immunosuppressed patients (e.g., HIV infection or transplant patients) and in those with congenital or perinatal infection, chronic CMV carriage for years is common without symptomatic disease. In such instances, isolation of CMV by itself does not necessarily suggest disease; demonstration of local pathology (by tissue biopsy or cytology) characteristics of CMV infection is often necessary.

## SUGGESTED READING

Ho M: Cytomegalovirus. In Mandell GL, Bennett JE, Dolin R, eds: *Principles and practices of infectious diseases,* ed 4, New York, 1995, Churchill Livingstone.

# Diverticulitis

Q How should diverticulitis be treated medically and surgically?

Most patients with acute diverticulitis require hospitalization. Occasionally a patient with minimal evidence of inflammation can be given a trial of an oral broad-spectrum antibiotic (see below for potential choices) and a liquid diet as an outpatient, but failure to improve after 48 hours dictates immediate admission to the hospital.

Inpatient therapy of acute diverticulitis should include bed rest, intravenous hydration and antibiotics, and bowel rest (nothing by mouth), particularly when nausea, vomiting, and abdominal distention are present; in cases associated with vomiting and abdominal distention, nasogastric tube decompression should also be considered. Excessive analgesia should be avoided to better monitor for progression of pain. Because of its propensity to increase colonic intraluminal pressure, the use of morphine sulfate should be avoided; meperidine hydrochloride should be considered instead.

Intravenous antibiotics should cover both the aerobic and anaerobic flora of the colon. Potential antibiotic choices include cefoxitin, cefotetan, ampicillin-sulbactam, ticarcillin/clavulanate, and piperacillin-tazobactam. Combinations of antibiotics such as an aminoglycoside (gentamicin or tobramycin) and either clindamycin or metronidazole, or ampicillin with gentamicin and either clindamycin or

**84**

metronidazole are also reasonable alternatives. In uncompli-cated diverticulitis, IV antibiotics should be continued until signs of toxicity, fever, and vomiting have resolved. Duration of antibiotic therapy is usually 7 to 10 days in uncomplicated cases. The majority of patients with diverticulitis improve with medical therapy and do not require surgery.

Although the indications for surgical intervention may vary from one medical institution to another, the following appear to be widely accepted:

1. Progressive symptoms or lack of improvement after 48 hours of medical therapy in the absence of an identifiable abscess on an abdominal/pelvis computed tomography (CT) scan or in the presence of an abscess not considered to be amenable to CT-guided drainage

2. Uncontrolled sepsis

3. Free viscus perforation

4. Uncontrolled fistulas

5. Bowel obstruction

6. Inflammatory involvement of the urinary tract

7. Inability to exclude colonic carcinoma

8. Two or more acute attacks of diverticulitis successfully treated medically

Although there is controversy regarding the need for surgery in patients younger than 40 years old (traditionally consid-ered to have more severe disease) following the first bout of diverticulitis, recent studies support the view that a single episode of diverticulitis in younger patients does not warrant an elective resection.

SUGGESTED READINGS

Ertan A: Colonic diverticulitis. Recognizing and managing its presentations and complications, *Postgrad Med* 88:67-72, 77, 1990.
Sanford JP, Gilbert DN, Sande MA: *Guide to antimicrobial therapy,* ed 26, Dallas, 1996, Antimicrobial Therapy.
Stabile BE: Therapeutic options in acute diverticulitis, *Compr Ther* 17:26-33, 1991.
Telford GL: Diverticulitis. In Fry DE, ed: *Surgical infections,* Boston, 1995, Little, Brown.
Vignati PV, Welch JP, Cohen JL: Long-term management of diverticulitis in young patients, *Dis Colon Rectum* 38:627-629, 1995.

 What are some choices of oral antibiotics for treatment of acute diverticulitis?

Oral antibiotics may be used for initial treatment of mild diverticulitis or following completion of IV therapy. As in the case of parenteral antibiotic treatment, coverage of coliform aerobic gram-negative bacilli and colonic anaerobes (e.g., *Bacteroides* sp.) is essential. A combination antibiotic such as amoxicillin/clavulanate (500 mg/125 mg 3×/day) is usually adequate. In penicillin-allergic patients, either trimethoprim-sulfamethoxazole 800 mg/160 mg (double strength) 2×/day or ciprofloxacin (500 mg 2×/day) *and* metronidazole 500 mg 4×/day is reasonable.

SUGGESTED READINGS

Sanford JP, Gilbert DN, Sande MA: *Guide to antimicrobial therapy,* ed 26, Dallas, 1996, Antimicrobial Therapy.
Stabile BE: Therapeutic options in acute diverticulitis, *Compr Ther* 17:26-33, 1991.

# Endocarditis

Q For which cardiac conditions is prophylaxis of bacterial endocarditis indicated?

The American Heart Association (AHA) recommends antibiotic prophylaxis for several cardiac conditions, including the following:

1. High-risk category (i.e., those at high risk for developing severe endocardial infection often associated with high morbidity and mortality):
    a. Prosthetic cardiac valves, including bioprosthetic and homograft valves
    b. Previous bacterial endocarditis, even in the absence of documented heart disease
    c. Complex cyanotic heart disease (e.g., single ventricle states, transposition of the great arteries, and Fallot's tetralogy)
    d. Surgically constructed systemic pulmonary shunts or conduits
2. Moderate-risk category (i.e., those at moderate risk for severe infection):
    a. Most other congenital cardiac malformations, including the following uncorrected conditions: patent ductus arteriosus, ventricular septal defect, primum atrial septal defect, coarctation of the aorta, and bicuspid aortic valve
    b. Acquired valvular dysfunction (e.g., caused by rheumatic heart disease or collagen vascular disease)

**87**

c. Hypertrophic cardiomyopathy

d. Mitral valve prolapse with valvular regurgitation or thickened leaflets (e.g., in the presence of murmur of mitral regurgitation, or echocardiographic Doppler demonstration of the same), or when presence or absence of mitral regurgitation is not determined or not known and there is immediate need for procedure; consider also for men older than 45 years with mitral valve prolapse, without a consistent systolic murmur, even in the absence of resting regurgitation

Antibiotic prophylaxis is *not* recommended by AHA for patients at *negligible risk* of severe infection (i.e., no greater risk than the general population):

1. Isolated secundum atrial septal defect

2. Surgical repair of atrial septal defect, ventricular septal defect, or patent ductus arteriosus (without residual beyond 6 months)

3. Previous coronary artery bypass graft surgery

4. Mitral valve prolapse without valvular regurgitation (see above)

5. Physiological, functional, or innocent heart murmurs

6. Previous Kawasaki disease without valvular dysfunction

7. Previous rheumatic fever without valvular dysfunction

8. Cardiac pacemakers (intravascular and epicardial) and implanted defibrillators

## ADDITIONAL CONSIDERATIONS

There is controversy regarding endocarditis prophylaxis in patients with mitral valve prolapse without regurgitation at rest. Because of the possibility of exercise-induced mitral regurgitation in as many as 33% of such patients, some have questioned the wisdom of giving antibiotic prophylaxis only to patients with regurgitation at rest.

Inflammatory bowel disease (e.g., ulcerative colitis and Crohn's disease) has been reported to be associated with higher risk of bacterial endocarditis. Antibiotic prophylaxis may need to be considered in patients with "highly active inflammatory bowel disease" even in the absence of cardiac factors predisposing to bacterial endocarditis.

### SUGGESTED READINGS

Cheng TO: Exercise-induced mitral regurgitation and antibiotic prophy-laxis against infective endocarditis in mitral valve prolapse [letter], *J Am Coll Cardiol* 26:839, 1995.

Dajani AS et al: Prevention of bacterial endocarditis: recommendations by the American Heart Association, *JAMA* 264:2919-2922, 1990.

Dajani AS et al: Prevention of bacterial endocarditis: recommendations by the American Heart Association, *JAMA* 277:1794-1801, 1997.

Kreuzpaintner G et al: Increased risk of bacterial endocarditis in inflam-matory bowel disease, *Am J Med* 92:391-395, 1992.

Uyemura MC: Antibiotic prophylaxis for medical and dental procedures: a look at AHA guidelines and controversial issues, *Postgrad Med* 98:137-154, 1995.

For which invasive procedures is endocarditis prophylaxis indicated?

AHA recommends endocarditis prophylaxis for several procedures, including the following:

1. Dental procedures associated with gingival or mucosal bleeding such as:
   a. Dental extractions
   b. Periodontal procedures including surgery, scaling and root planing, probing, and recall maintenance
   c. Dental implant placement and reimplantation of avulsed teeth
   d. Endodontic (root canal) instrumentation or surgery only beyond the apex
   e. Subgingival placement of antibiotic fibers or strips
   f. Initial placement of orthodontic bands but not brackets
   g. Intraligamentary local anesthetic injections
   h. Prophylactic cleaning of teeth or implants where bleeding is anticipated
2. Respiratory tract procedures including:
   a. Tonsillectomy or adenoidectomy
   b. Surgical operations that involve respiratory mucosa
   c. Bronchoscopy with a rigid bronchoscope
   d. Optional in high-risk patients only: bronchoscopy with a flexible bronchoscope with or without biopsy
3. Gastrointestinal tract procedures (recommended for high-risk patients; optional for medium-risk patients) including:
   a. Sclerotherapy or esophageal varices
   b. Esophageal stricture dilation
   c. Endoscopic retrograde cholangiography with biliary obstruction
   d. Biliary tract surgery
   e. Surgical operations that involve intestinal mucosa

    f. Optional in high-risk patients only: transesophageal echocardiography and endoscopy with or without gastrointestinal biopsy

4. Genitourinary tract procedures including:
    a. Prostatic surgery
    b. Cystoscopy
    c. Urethral dilation
    d. Optional in high-risk patients only: vaginal hysterectomy and vaginal delivery

In addition to the AHA guidelines previously listed, the question of expanding endocarditis prophylaxis to include several other procedures has been raised in the literature. These *suggestions* should be considered only on a case-by-case basis and should not be construed as "standard of care."

1. Dermatological surgical manipulation of eroded, noninfected skin in AHA "high-risk" patients (with prosthetic valve)

2. Dermatological surgical manipulation involving large incision requiring more than 20 minutes to close in AHA "high-risk" patients (with prosthetic valve)

3. Women who deliver by cesarean section after labor

SUGGESTED READINGS

Anonymous: Antibiotic prophylaxis for gastrointestinal endoscopy, *Gastrointest Endo* 42:630-635, 1995.

Boggess KA et al: Bacteremia shortly after placental separation during cesarean delivery, *Obstet Gynecol* 87:779-784, 1996.

Dajani AS et al: Prevention of bacterial endocarditis: recommendations by the American Heart Association, *JAMA* 264:2919-2922, 1990.

Dajani AS et al: Prevention of bacterial endocarditis: recommendations by the American Heart Association, *JAMA* 277:1794-1801, 1997.

Haas AF, Grekin RC: Antibiotic prophylaxis in dermatologic surgery, *J Am Acad Dermatol* 32:155-176, 1995.

For what procedures is bacterial endocarditis prophylaxis *not* recommended?

1. Certain dental procedures not associated with significant bleeding, including:
   a. Restorative dentistry (operative and prosthodontic, filling cavities, and replacement of missing teeth) with or without retraction cord (except in circumstances associated with significant bleeding)
   b. Local anesthetic injections (nonintraligamentary)
   c. Intracanal endodontic treatment; postplacement and buildup
   d. Placement of rubber dams
   e. Postoperative suture removal
   f. Placement of removable prosthodontic or orthodontic appliances
   g. Taking of oral impressions
   h. Fluoride treatments
   i. Taking of oral radiographs
   j. Orthodontic appliance adjustment
   k. Shedding of primary teeth
2. Respiratory tract procedures including:
   a. Endotracheal intubation
   b. Bronchoscopy with a flexible bronchoscope with or without biopsy (optional for high-risk patients)
   c. Tympanostomy tube insertion
3. Gastrointestinal tract:
   a. Transesophageal echocardiography (optional for high-risk patients)
   b. Endoscopy with or without gastrointestinal biopsy (optional for high-risk patients)
4. Genitourinary tract:
   a. Vaginal hysterectomy (optional for high-risk patients)
   b. Vaginal delivery (optional for high-risk patients)

   c. Cesarean section
   d. In uninfected tissue:
- Urethral catheterization
- Uterine dilation and curettage
- Therapeutic abortion
- Sterilization procedures
- Insertion or removal of intrauterine devices

5. Miscellaneous:
   a. Cardiac catheterization, including balloon angioplasty
   b. Implanted cardiac devices, including:
- Pacemakers
- Defibrillators
- Coronary stents

   c. Incision or biopsy of surgically scrubbed skin
   d. Circumcision

## ADDITIONAL CONSIDERATIONS

1. When unanticipated bleeding occurs during dental procedures not requiring prophylaxis, antimicrobial administration within 2 hours following the procedure may be effective (based on experimental animal data); antibiotic administration more than 4 hours after the procedure will probably not have any value.

2. Prophylaxis is also recommended for any other genitourinary tract procedure (not previously listed) in the presence of infection.

### SUGGESTED READING
Dajani AS et al: Prevention of bacterial endocarditis: recommendations by the American Heart Association, *JAMA* 277:1794-1801, 1997.

Is bacterial endocarditis prophylaxis necessary for clean surgical procedures involving joints, including arthroplasty and arthroscopy?

Clean surgical procedures not involving the respiratory, gastrointestinal, and genitourinary tracts are not associated with high risk of bacteremia and, therefore, should not require endocarditis prophylaxis.

**SUGGESTED READING**

Dajani AS et al: Prevention of bacterial endocarditis: recommendations by the American Heart Association, *JAMA* 277:1794-1801, 1997.

 What antibiotics may be used for bacterial endocarditis prophylaxis?

AHA recommends the following antibiotic regimen for endocarditis prophylaxis. The selection of antibiotic prophylaxis is contingent on the presence or absence of penicillin allergy, risk status of the patient, and the type of procedure planned.

## PATIENTS WITH NO PENICILLIN ALLERGY

Patients undergoing dental, oral, upper respiratory tract, or esophageal procedures:

Adults: amoxicillin 2 g
Children: 50 mg/kg PO 1 hr before procedure
*If unable to take oral medications:*
Adults: ampicillin 2 g IM or IV
Children: 50 mg/kg IM or IV; administered within 30 min of starting the procedure

Patients considered high risk (see p. 87 for definition) and undergoing genitourinary or gastrointestinal (excluding esophageal) procedures:

Adults: ampicillin 2 g IM or IV and gentamicin 1.5 mg/kg (maximum 120 mg) within 30 min of starting the procedure; 6 hrs later, ampicillin 1 g IM or IV or amoxicillin 1 g PO
Children: ampicillin 50 mg/kg IM or IV (maximum 2 g) and gentamicin 1.5 mg/kg within 30 min of starting the procedure; 6 hrs later, ampicillin 25 mg/kg IM or IV or amoxicillin 25 mg/kg PO

Patients considered moderate risk (see pp. 87 to 88 for definition) and undergoing genitourinary/gastrointestinal (excluding esophageal) procedures:

Adults: amoxicillin 2 g PO 1 hr before procedure or ampicillin 2 g IM or IV within 30 min of starting the procedure
Children: amoxicillin 50 mg/kg PO 1 hr before procedure or ampicillin 50 mg/kg IM or IV within 30 min of starting the procedure

## PATIENTS WITH PENICILLIN ALLERGY
Patients undergoing dental, oral, respiratory tract, or esophageal procedures:

Adults: clindamycin 600 mg PO 1 hr before procedure or cephalexin or cefadroxil 2 g PO 1 hr before procedure or azithromycin or clarithromycin 500 mg 1 hr before procedure
Adults unable to take PO medications: clindamycin 600 mg IV within 30 min of starting the procedure or cefazolin (in the absence of immediate hypersensitivity-type reaction to penicillins) 1 g IV within 30 min before procedure
Children: clindamycin 20 mg/kg (maximum 600 mg) PO 1 hr before procedure or cephalexin or cefadroxil 50 mg/kg

(maximum 2 g) PO 1 hr before procedure or azithromycin or clarithromycin 15 mg/kg (maximum 500 mg) orally 1 hr before procedure

Children unable to take PO medications: clindamycin 20 mg/kg (maximum 600 mg) IV within 30 min of starting the procedure or cefazolin (in the absence of immediate-type hypersensitivity reaction to penicillins) 25 mg/kg (maximum 1 g) IM or IV within 30 min of starting the procedure

Patients considered high risk (see p. 87 for definition) and undergoing genitourinary or gastrointestinal (excluding esophageal) procedures:

Adults: vancomycin 1 g IV over 1 to 2 hrs and gentamicin 1.5 mg/kg IV or IM (maximum 120 mg); complete injection/ infusion within 30 min of starting the procedure

Children: vancomycin 20 mg/kg IV (maximum 1 g) over 1 to 2 hrs and gentamicin 1.5 mg/kg (maximum 120 mg) IV or IM; complete injection/infusion within 30 min of starting the procedure

Patients considered to be at moderate risk (see pp. 87 to 88 for definition) and undergoing genitourinary or gastrointestinal (excluding esophageal) procedures:

Adults: vancomycin 1 g IV over 1 to 2 hrs; complete infusion within 30 min of starting the procedure

Children: vancomycin 20 mg/kg IV (maximum 1 g) over 1 to 2 hrs; complete infusion within 30 minutes of starting the procedure

## ADDITIONAL CONSIDERATIONS

1. AHA no longer recommends erythromycin as an alternative agent in patients with penicillin allergy because of gastrointestinal upset and complicated pharmacokinetics of the

various formulations. However, practitioners who have successfully used erythromycin for prophylaxis in individual patients may choose to continue with this antibiotic.

2. Tetracycline and sulfonamides are not recommended for endocarditis prophylaxis.

3. Antibiotics used to prevent the recurrence of acute rheumatic fever are inadequate for the prevention of bacterial endocarditis. Patients using chronic oral penicillin for secondary prevention of rheumatic fever or other conditions may have streptococci in their oral cavities that are relatively resistant to penicillin, amoxicillin, or ampicillin. In such cases alternative antibiotics such as clindamycin, azithromycin, or clarithromycin should be used.

4. Follow-up dose after the procedure is no longer recommended except for high-risk patients undergoing genitourinary or gastrointestinal (excluding esophageal) procedures and receiving ampicillin IV (revised AHA recommendation, 1997).

5. When a series of dental procedures is anticipated, it is reasonable to allow an interval of 9 to 14 days between procedures to allow repopulation of oral cavity with antibiotic-susceptible flora.

6. In patients who receive heparin, IM injections for endocarditis prophylaxis should be avoided; use of warfarin sodium is a relative contraindication to IM injections. In these settings, IV or PO regimens should be used whenever possible.

7. Good oral hygiene may be more effective in preventing infective endocarditis than antibiotics. Brushing, flossing, and the use of fluoride rinses and antiseptic mouthwashes before dental procedures are recommended.

SUGGESTED READINGS

Dajani AS et al: Prevention of bacterial endocarditis: recommendations by the American Heart Association, *JAMA* 264:2919-2922, 1990.

Dajani AS et al: Prevention of bacterial endocarditis: recommendations by the American Heart Association, *JAMA* 277:1794-1801, 1997.

Uyemura MC: Antibiotic prophylaxis for medical and dental procedures: a look at AHA guidelines and controversial issues, *Postgrad Med* 98:137-154, 1995.

## STIMULATING QUESTION

Is bacterial endocarditis prophylaxis necessary before rectal examination?

Even with more invasive procedures such as sigmoidoscopy and colonoscopy, antibiotic prophylaxis is not routinely recommended. Therefore prophylaxis before rectal examination is not necessary.

SUGGESTED READINGS

Anonymous: Antibiotic prophylaxis for gastrointestinal endoscopy, *Gastrointest Endosc* 42:630-635, 1995.

Dajani AS et al: Prevention of bacterial endocarditis: recommendations by the American Heart Association, *JAMA* 264:2919-2922, 1990.

Dajani AS et al: Prevention of bacterial endocarditis: recommendations by the American Heart Association, *JAMA* 277:1794-1801, 1997.

## STIMULATING QUESTION

Why was amoxicillin (rather than penicillin) chosen for bacterial endocarditis prophylaxis, and is repeat dosing after 6 hours necessary?

Although amoxicillin, ampicillin, and penicillin V have comparable activity in vitro against viridans streptococci, amoxicillin is now recommended because of its enhanced absorption from the gastrointestinal tract and achievement of higher and more sustained serum levels.

A recent study of serum drug levels after 3-g and 2-g doses of oral amoxicillin in healthy adults has demonstrated that a single 2-g dose of this antibiotic achieves adequate serum levels for at least 6 hours after administration of the dose. Therefore, for prevention of bacterial endocarditis, a single 2-g dose of oral amoxicillin may be adequate prophylaxis for dental, oral, or upper respiratory tract procedures; this regimen was recently adopted by the AHA (1997).

## SUGGESTED READINGS

Dajani AS, Bawdon RE, Berry MC: Oral amoxicillin as prophylaxis for endocarditis: what is the optimal dose? *Clin Infect Dis* 18:157-160, 1994.

Dajani AS et al: Prevention of bacterial endocarditis: recommendations by the American Heart Association, *JAMA* 264:2919-2922, 1990.

Dajani AS et al: Prevention of bacterial endocarditis: recommendations by the American Heart Association, *JAMA* 277:1794-1801, 1997.

# Enterococcus

What antibiotic(s) should be used for treatment of enterococcal bacteremia, endocarditis, urinary tract infection, or wound infection? Is combination therapy including an aminoglycoside always necessary?

Enterococci *(Enterococcus faecalis* and *Enterococcus faecium)* are commonly resistant to clinically achievable levels of cephalosporins, clindamycin, nafcillin, oxacillin, and aminoglycosides and are relatively resistant to carbenicillin and ticarcillin. Imipenem and ciprofloxacin may also be active against certain strains. *Penicillin/ampicillin and vancomycin are the drugs of choice for treatment of infections caused by susceptible enterococci, but neither alone is bactericidal against these organisms.* In vitro activity of piperacillin and mezlocillin against enterococci approaches that of penicillin. In clinical situations in which a bactericidal effect is desired (e.g., endocarditis, sepsis in granulocytopenic host, and possibly meningitis or osteomyelitis), an aminoglycoside toward which the isolate does not demonstrate high-level resistance should be used in combination with penicillin/ampicillin or vancomycin.

Enterococcal bacteremia without endocarditis may be treated with an active agent (e.g., penicillin/ampicillin or vancomycin) alone in nongranulocytopenic hosts. Duration of therapy is usually 10 to 14 days.

Enterococcal endocarditis is commonly treated with an active agent (e.g., penicillin/ampicillin or vancomycin) and

**100**

an aminoglycoside (usually gentamicin). It should be noted that the desired peak aminoglycoside level is much lower than that aimed for gram-negative infections because of the use of the aminoglycoside as a "synergistic drug." As such, peak levels of 3 to 5 μg/ml are usually considered adequate in this setting. Duration of therapy is usually 4 to 6 weeks.

Enterococcal urinary tract infection without bacteremia or signs of sepsis can often be treated with oral antibiotics alone such as ampicillin, nitrofurantoin, or a quinolone (e.g., ciprofloxacin), assuming in vitro susceptibility to these drugs.

Enterococcal wound infection is often found in association with infection caused by other organisms, and specific treatment of this organism may not be necessary, depending on the clinical situation (e.g., in the absence of bacteremia, clinical evidence of infection, or purulent discharge). When therapy is desired, use of ampicillin/penicillin, piperacillin, mezlocillin, or vancomycin should be considered. Duration of treatment should be based on clinical picture, but a 7- to 10-day course of treatment is reasonable.

Recent emergence of vancomycin-resistant enterococcal isolates has made treatment of these organisms even more problematic. Treatment should be based on in vitro susceptibility. Chloramphenicol (500 to 1000 mg every 6 to 8 hrs, IV or PO) may be effective in the treatment of serious vancomycin-resistant enterococcal infections. An experimental drug, quinupristin/dalfopristin (Synercid) possesses in vitro inhibitory and bactericidal activity against many strains of vancomycin-resistant *E. faecium,* but its clinical efficacy has not yet been fully evaluated.

## SUGGESTED READINGS

Chant C, Rybak MJ: Quinupristin/dalfopristin (RP 59500): a new streptogramin antibiotic, *Ann Parmacother* 29:1022-1027, 1995.
Maki DG, Agger WA: Enterococcal bacteremia: clinical features, the risk of endocarditis, and management, *Medicine* 67:248-269, 1988.

Norris AH et al: Chloramphenicol for the treatment of vancomycin-resistant enterococcal infections, *Clin Infect Dis* 20:1137-1144, 1995.

Tailor SA, Bailey EM, Rybak MJ: *Enterococcus,* an emerging pathogen, *Ann Pharmacother* 27:1231-1242, 1993.

What isolation precautions should be used in the care of hospitalized patients with vancomycin-resistant enterococcal infections?

The Hospital Infection Control Practices Advisory Committee (HICPAC) recommends "contact precautions." In addition to standard precautions, the patient is placed in a private room whenever possible or placed in a room with another patient with vancomycin-resistant enterococcal colonization or infection (cohorting). Gloves should be worn when entering the room and removed before leaving the patient's room. Gowns should be worn when entering the room if substantial contact with the patient, environmental surfaces, or items in the patient's room is anticipated or if the patient is incontinent or has diarrhea, an ileostomy or colostomy, or wound drainage not contained by a dressing. Transport of patient outside of the room should be minimized. When the use of noncritical patient-care equipment or items is unavoidable, they should be adequately cleansed and disinfected before their use on another patient.

**SUGGESTED READING**

Garner JS: Guidelines for isolation precautions in hospitals, *Infect Control Hosp Epidemiol* 17:53-80, 1996.

# Epstein-Barr Virus

 How should Epstein-Barr virus (EBV) serologies be interpreted?

There are two basic serological tests for EBV infection: non-specific (heterophile) and specific antibody tests. Paul-Bunnell, or rapid heterophile antibody slide agglutination, test (monospot) may take 3 to 5 days (range 0 to 21 days) to become positive following onset of symptoms, peaks during the second week of illness (range 1 to 4 weeks), and usually becomes negative in 2 to 3 months (may persist at 1 year in 20% of cases). False-positive results have been associated with lymphoma or hepatitis.

Testing for EBV-specific antibodies is usually not necessary unless monospot antibody is undetectable in a suspected or atypical case or to help exclude false-positive monospot test. EBV viral capsid antibody (VCA) IgM is present in virtually all cases of acute mononucleosis (97% sensitive, 99% specific) at the time of presentation and usually persists for 4 to 8 weeks. EBV VCA IgG is also present in all cases of acute mononucleosis and persists lifelong. Epstein-Barr nucleic acid (EBNA) antibody usually is present 3 to 4 weeks after onset of illness ("late" antibody) and persists lifelong; conversion from negative to a positive EBNA antibody test supports a diagnosis of recent EBV infection.

## SUGGESTED READINGS

Evans AS et al: A prospective evaluation of heterophile and Epstein-Barr virus–specific IgM antibody tests in clinical and subclinical infectious mononucleosis: specificity and sensitivity of the tests and persistence of antibody, *J Infect Dis* 132:546-554, 1975.

Schooley RT: Epstein-Barr virus (infectious mononucleosis). In Mandell GL, Bennett JE, Dolin R, eds: *Principles and practices of infectious diseases,* ed 4, New York, 1995, Churchill Livingstone.

 Is there a role for testing for EBV antibodies in the evaluation of patients with chronic fatigue?

By adulthood, 90% to 95% of most populations have demonstrable EBV antibodies. One study reported elevation of EBV VCA IgG antibody at 1:320 titers or greater in 15% of age- and gender-matched healthy adults compared with 55% of patients with chronic fatigue syndrome (CFS). EBV VCA titers of 1:640 or greater may be found in 5% of healthy adults and 45% of patients with CFS. Attempts at documenting higher viral shedding or load in body fluids of CFS patients compared with healthy controls have been unsuccessful. These findings, along with the generally nonspecific nature of elevated EBV VCA IgG antibody titers (i.e., may be elevated in other conditions), render interpretation of this antibody test in individual patients with fatigue difficult and diagnostically not useful.

## SUGGESTED READINGS

Jones JF: Serologic and immunologic responses in chronic fatigue syndrome with emphasis on the Epstein-Barr virus, *Rev Infect Dis* 13(suppl 1):S26-S31, 1991.

Manian FA: Simultaneous measurement of antibodies to Epstein-Barr virus, human herpesvirus 6, herpes simplex virus types 1 and 2, and 14 enteroviruses in chronic fatigue syndrome: is there evidence of activation of a nonspecific polyclonal immune response? *Clin Infect Dis* 19:448-453, 1994.

Matthews DA, Lane TJ, Manu P: Antibodies to Epstein-Barr virus in patients with chronic fatigue, *South Med J* 84:832-840, 1991.

Schooley RT: Epstein-Barr virus (infectious mononucleosis). In Mandell GL, Bennett JE, Dolin R, eds: *Principles and practices of infectious diseases,* ed 4, New York, 1995, Churchill Livingstone.

Swanink CM et al: Epstein-Barr virus (EBV) and the chronic fatigue syndrome: normal virus load in blood and normal immunologic reactivity in the EBV regression assay, *Clin Infect Dis* 20:1390-1392, 1995.

 How should EBV mononucleosis be managed? Is there a role for antiviral therapy?

The majority of patients with EBV mononucleosis (greater than 95%) will recover uneventfully without specific therapy.

General recommendations for the care of such patients include the following:

1. Tailor activity level as tolerated by the patient. Many patients require extended amount of rest and sleep, particularly during the early phase of the illness.
2. Contact sports or heavy lifting should be avoided at least during the first 2 to 3 weeks of illness, particularly when splenomegaly is present.
3. Sore throat may be alleviated by acetaminophen, aspirin, or ibuprofen and by gargling with warm salt water.
4. Fever (often lasting 10 to 14 days) may be treated or suppressed by the use of acetaminophen, aspirin, or ibuprofen.
5. Constipation, when present, should be treated with a gentle laxative.
6. Corticosteroid use generally decreases the period of febrility and helps resolve many constitutional symptoms; however, their use in uncomplicated EBV mononucleosis

remains controversial. They should be considered in the following settings:

a. Impending airway obstruction
b. Severe thrombocytopenia
c. Hemolytic anemia
d. CNS involvement
e. Myocarditis
f. Pericarditis
g. Severe or prolonged prostration

The usual dose of prednisone is 60 to 80 mg/day given in divided daily regimen, with tapering doses over a 1- to 2-week period; tapering over a longer period may be indicated in patients with severe or prolonged prostration.

7. Use of acyclovir (oral or parenteral) in EBV mononucleosis has been associated with inhibition of viral shedding from the oropharynx. *However, acyclovir has not demonstrated sufficient clinical benefit to recommend its use in the setting of uncomplicated disease.* Its use in complicated EBV mononucleosis has not been adequately studied.

8. Combined use of acyclovir and prednisolone has also been shown not to have any impact on the duration of clinical symptoms, sore throat, weight loss, or absence from school or work.

SUGGESTED READINGS

Bailey RE: Diagnosis and treatment of infectious mononucleosis, *Am Fam Physician* 49:879-888, 1994.

Schooley RT: Epstein-Barr virus (infectious mononucleosis). In Mandell GL, Bennett JE, Dolin R, eds: *Principles and practices of infectious diseases,* ed 4, New York, 1995, Churchill Livingstone.

Tynell E et al: Acyclovir and prednisolone treatment of acute infectious mononucleosis: a multicenter, double-blind, placebo-controlled study, *J Infect Dis* 174:324-331, 1996.

Van der Horst et al: Lack of effect of peroral acyclovir for the treatment of acute infectious mononucleosis, *J Infect Dis* 164:788-792, 1991.

# Gastroenteritis

 What is the best way to prevent and treat traveler's diarrhea?

Traveler's diarrhea is acquired through ingestion of fecally contaminated food (e.g., raw or undercooked meat and seafood, unpasteurized milk and dairy products, or raw vegetables and fruits), water (e.g., tap water), and ice. Bottled water, carbonated beverages (especially flavored beverages), beer, wine, hot coffee or tea, and treated water (boiled or appropriately treated with iodine or chlorine) are considered safe. The most important risk factor for traveler's diarrhea is the destination of the traveler (highest risk areas include most of the developing countries of Latin America, Africa, the Middle East, and Asia). The place of food preparation is also an important factor, with private homes, restaurants, and street vendors listed in order of increasing risk. Meticulous attention to food and beverage consumption can decrease the likelihood of developing traveler's diarrhea.

Prophylactic use of bismuth subsalicylate (Pepto-Bismol, 2 oz or 2 tablets 4×/day) can decrease the incidence of diarrhea by 60% but is not recommended for periods of more than 3 weeks and should be avoided in patients who are allergic to salicylates or taking salicylates or anticoagulants. Prophylactic antimicrobial agents are not routinely recommended for prevention of traveler's diarrhea because of uncertain risk of widespread administration of antibiotics and their potential for causing adverse reactions in travelers (e.g., allergic, antibi-

**107**

otic-associated colitis; photosensitivity; blood disorders; or *Candida* vaginitis). It may be reasonable to consider the use of prophylactic antibiotics (e.g., ciprofloxacin 500 mg/day, ofloxacin 300 mg/day, or norfloxacin 400 mg/day) in certain high-risk groups such as travelers with immunosuppression or immunodeficiency.

Travelers who develop diarrhea with three or more loose stools in an 8-hour period, particularly when associated with nausea, vomiting, abdominal cramps, fever, or blood in the stools, may benefit from antimicrobial therapy: ciprofloxacin 500 mg 2×/day, norfloxacin 400 mg 2×/day, or ofloxacin 300 mg 2×/day for no more than 3 days in adults. Trimethoprim-sulfamethoxazole 160/800 mg 2×/day can be used for children, but resistance is common in many areas. Antimotility agents such as loperamide (Imodium) and diphenoxylate (Lomotil) should not be used in patients with high fever or blood in stool, when symptoms last beyond 48 hours, or in children less than 2 years of age. Packets of oral rehydration salts available in the United States (Cera Products, Columbia, Md, 410-997-2334; Jianas Brothers, Kansas City, Mo, 816-421-2880) and in stores and pharmacies in many developing countries may be added to boiled or treated water to help replace fluids and salts; once solution is prepared it should be consumed or discarded within 12 hours if held at room temperature or 24 hours if held refrigerated.

## SUGGESTED READINGS

Anonymous: Advice for travelers, *Med Lett Drugs Ther* 38:17-20, 1996.
Centers for Disease Control and Prevention, US Department of Health and Human Services: *Health information for international travel* 1996-1997, Washington, DC, December 1996, US Government Printing Office.

Should *Blastocystis hominis* in stool be treated?

Although for many years *B. hominis* was considered a potential pathogen causing diarrhea, recent clinical studies have overwhelmingly questioned the pathogenicity of this organism, even in severely immunocompromised hosts. Similar rates of *B. hominis* detection in stools of travelers with diarrhea and those of asymptomatic controls (30% vs. 36%, respectively) have been reported. High prevalence of concurrent infection with other protozoa (e.g., *Giardia* and *Entamoeba histolytica)* supports the need to exclude the presence of these pathogens when *B. hominis* is found in stool of patients with diarrhea. Although iodoquinol and metronidazole have in vitro activity against *B. hominis,* there is generally *no* reason to treat *Blastocystis* infections.

## SUGGESTED READINGS

Keystone JS: *Blastocystis hominis* and traveler's diarrhea, *Clin Infect Dis* 21:102-103, 1995 (editorial).
Markell EK: Is there any reason to continue treating *Blastocystis* infections? *Clin Infect Dis* 21:104-105, 1995 (editorial).
Shlim DR et al: Is *Blastocystis hominis* a cause of diarrhea in travelers? A prospective controlled study in Nepal, *Clin Infect Dis* 21:97-101, 1995.

 How and in whom should *Salmonella* gastroenteritis be treated?

In normal hosts, *Salmonella* gastroenteritis is usually a self-limited disease; therefore the primary treatment involves fluid and electrolyte replacement. The use of opiates to decrease bowel motility in this condition is not recommended because of the possibility of increasing the incidence and extent of bacteremia.

Antibiotic treatment of uncomplicated *Salmonella* gastroenteritis does not appear to dramatically improve symptoms or outcome and may, in fact, be associated with higher bacteriological relapse rates. However, antibiotic therapy is indicated for those with continuous or high fever, manifestations of extraintestinal infection, or one of the following risk factors for development of severe complications following transient bacteremia: (1) newborn age, because of high risk of meningitis; (2) greater than 50 years of age, because of the high risk of infecting atherosclerotic plaques and aneurysms; (3) lymphoproliferative disorders; (4) suspected or known anatomical cardiovascular disease; (5) significant bone or joint disease, including the presence of a prosthesis or a foreign body; (6) sickle-cell disease or other forms of chronic hemolysis; (7) organ transplant; and (8) HIV infection, particularly with AIDS.

Antibiotic selection should be based on in vitro susceptibility data whenever possible. Third-generation cephalosporins (e.g., ceftriaxone), quinolones (e.g., ciprofloxacin), aztreonam, trimethoprim-sulfamethoxazole, and amoxicillin are potential choices. The first- and second-generation cephalosporins and the aminoglycosides should be avoided because of lack of clinical efficacy.

### SUGGESTED READINGS

Goldberg MB, Rubin RH: Nontyphoidal *Salmonella* infection. In Gorbach SL, Bartlett JG, Blacklow NR, eds: *Infectious diseases,* Philadelphia, 1992, WB Saunders.

Miller SI, Hohman EL, Pegues DA: *Salmonella* (including *Salmonella typhi).* In Mandell GL, Bennett JE, Dolin R, eds: *Principles and practices of infectious diseases,* ed 4, New York, 1995, Churchill Livingstone.

## STIMULATING QUESTION

Should immunocompetent patients with cryptosporidial diarrhea be treated?

Cryptosporidial diarrhea in immunocompetent or temporarily immunocompromised patients is self-limited and requires symptomatic treatment only.

### SUGGESTED READING

Ungar BLP: Cryptosporidium. In Mandell GL, Bennett JE, Dolin R, eds: *Principles and practices of infectious diseases,* New York, 1995, Churchill Livingstone.

# Hepatitis A

 For whom and how should hepatitis A prophylaxis be administered?

There are two approaches to prophylaxis of hepatitis A: passive immunization with the use of immunoglobulin and active immunization with the use of the vaccine.

Immunoglobulin (IG) administration is indicated in the following circumstances:

1. Preexposure (e.g., susceptible travelers to developing countries)
2. Postexposure
   a. Close personal contact (e.g., all household and sexual contacts of persons with hepatitis A)
   b. Day care center (e.g., all staff and attendees of day care centers attended by children in diapers if one or more children or employees are diagnosed to have hepatitis A or if cases are diagnosed in two or more households of center attendees)
   c. Classroom-centered outbreak in schools; routine IG prophylaxis for pupils or teachers in contact with a patient is not indicated
   d. Hospitals (e.g., persons exposed to feces of infected patients); routine IG prophylaxis for hospital personnel is not indicated
   e. Common-source exposure (e.g., those involving food or water); IG prophylaxis is indicated for co-workers

112

of food handlers with hepatitis A but is usually not indicated for patrons unless all of the following conditions exist:

- The infected person is directly involved in handling foods, without gloves, that will not be cooked before they are eaten
- The hygienic practices of the food handler are suboptimal or the food handler has had diarrhea
- Patrons can be identified and offered prophylaxis within 2 weeks of exposure

The dose of IG is usually 0.02 ml/kg to 2 ml as a single IM injection. When preexposure prophylaxis of greater than 3 months is desired (e.g., certain travelers), 0.06 ml/kg to 5 ml is usually given. In the setting of postexposure prophylaxis, IG should be administered within 2 weeks of exposure.

## ACTIVE IMMUNIZATION/VACCINATION

Two recently released inactivated hepatitis A vaccines (Havrix and Vaqta) have been shown to be highly effective in preventing hepatitis A disease in persons 2 years of age and older. Havrix dose for adults is 1 ml (1440 U) IM in the deltoid, with a second dose in 6 to 12 months. For children 2 to 18 years, 0.5 ml (720 U) of Havrix is given at the same schedule as adults; alternatively, 360 U per 0.5 ml is given at 0, 1, and 6 to 12 months. Dosing of Vaqta is similar to that of Havrix (see package insert).

Havrix produces protective levels of antibodies against hepatitis A in 70% of recipients at 14 days and in more than 95% at 1 month after vaccination. Vaqta has been shown to produce protective levels of antibody at 4 weeks after a single dose in 90% to 99% of children 2 to 16 years old and adults who weigh less than 77 kg (170 lb). The efficacy of the vaccines in preventing clinical hepatitis A is 94% to 100%; their efficacy in preventing disease after exposure to hepatitis A has not been well studied. For those requiring combined immediate and long-term protection, vaccine may be given concomitantly with IG using separate sites and syringes.

*Hepatitis A vaccine is recommended for the following persons:* travelers to countries in which the hepatitis A virus is endemic, children in communities with high rates of hepatitis A, men who have sex with men, illicit drug users, patients with chronic liver disease, persons who work with primates that are infected with hepatitis A virus or work with this virus in a research setting, and persons with clotting factor disorders. Vaccination may also be considered for day care workers, food handlers, and the staff of institutions for the developmentally challenged. Hepatitis A vaccine is not routinely recommended for health care workers.

Prevaccination serological testing is considered most cost-effective in high-risk populations (e.g., previously mentioned groups and those born in countries with high endemicity of hepatitis A) and in persons over 40 years of age. Postvaccination serological testing is not recommended because of the high immunogenicity of the vaccine.

## SUGGESTED READINGS

Battlegay M, Gust ID, Feinstone SM: Hepatitis A virus. In Mandell GL, Bennett JE, Dolin R, eds: *Principles and practices of infectious diseases,* ed 4, New York, 1995, Churchill Livingstone.

Centers for Disease Control and Prevention: Licensure of inactivated hepatitis A vaccine and recommendations for use among international travelers, *MMWR* 44:559-560, 1995.

Gardner P et al: Adult immunizations, *Ann Intern Med* 12:35-40, 1996.

Moyer L, Warwick M, Mahoney FJ: Prevention of hepatitis A virus infection, *Am Fam Physician* 54:107-114, 1996.

## STIMULATING QUESTION

A health care worker was stuck by a needle contaminated by the blood of a patient who has acute hepatitis A. Is IG administration indicated?

Hepatitis A is usually transmitted by fecal-oral route. However, because hepatitis A viremia occurs during the prodromal phase of the disease, rarely, asymptomatic blood donors have been the source of infection by transfusion. If the source patient is already symptomatic from hepatitis A, it is unlikely that he or she is viremic at the time of the exposure. When viremia occurs, it is associated with low viral concentration in the blood. For these reasons, hepatitis A transmission by needle-stick injury would be unlikely and has not been reported to date. Nevertheless, immune serum globulin may be administered (similar to that used for postexposure prophylaxis; see previous discussion) if there is any lingering concern over the potential transmission of hepatitis A in this setting.

### SUGGESTED READINGS

Battlegay M, Gust ID, Feinstone SM: Hepatitis A virus. In Mandell GL, Bennett JE, Dolin R, eds: *Principles and practices of infectious diseases,* ed 4, New York, 1995, Churchill Livingstone.

Centers for Disease Control and Prevention: Hepatitis A among persons with hemophilia who received clotting factor concentrate—United States, September-December 1995, *MMWR* 45:29-32, 1996.

## STIMULATING QUESTION

Can a person who recently received immune serum globulin or vaccine products donate blood?

As long as the donor is asymptomatic, he or she may donate blood after receiving immune serum globulin.

Persons who have recently received toxoids and killed viral, bacterial, and rickettsial vaccines may donate blood as long as they are asymptomatic and afebrile. These include but are not limited to vaccines against cholera, diphtheria, hepatitis A, hepatitis B, influenza, pertussis, plague, polio (injectable, Salk), paratyphoid, Rocky Mountain spotted fever (RMSF), tetanus, typhoid, and typhus. Persons who have received human diploid cell rabies vaccine are also accepted if they are asymptomatic and afebrile unless the vaccination has been given following an animal bite, in which case the donor is deferred for 1 year after the bite.

Persons who have received live attenuated viral vaccines such as rubeola (measles) (within 2 weeks), rubella (German measles) (within 4 weeks), mumps (within 2 weeks), yellow fever (within 2 weeks), or oral polio vaccine (within 2 weeks) should be deferred. Those receiving hepatitis B immmune globulin should be deferred for 12 months.

### SUGGESTED READING

Standards Committee of the American Association of Blood Banks: *Donor selection for allogeneic blood. Standards for blood banks and transfusion services,* ed 17, Bethesda, Md, 1996, American Association of Blood Banks.

# Hepatitis B

 *Q* How should hepatitis B virus (HBV) serological tests be interpreted?

1. Hepatitis B surface antigen (HbsAg) + , hepatitis B core antibody (HbcAb) − : up to 17% of patients with early-stage acute HBV infection may have this profile.

2. HbsAg +, HbcAb +, hepatitis B surface antibody (HbsAb) −: may be seen in acute infection and in chronic HBV carriage with or without symptoms.

3. HbsAg −, HbcAb +, HbsAb −: "window" period of acute infection (before HbsAb develops but after HbsAg disappears), chronic HBV infection with HbsAg below threshold for detection by available tests, old HBV infection, and false-positive (particularly in blood donors).

Note: *The presence of HbcAb IgM favors a recent or acute infection.*

4. HbsAg −, HbcAb +, HbsAb +: prior HBV infection with recovery.

5. HbsAg −, HbcAb −, HbsAb +: recent hepatitis B vaccination, old infection.

SUGGESTED READINGS

Ravel R: *Clinical laboratory medicine,* ed 6, St Louis, 1995, Mosby.
Robinson WS: Hepatitis B virus and hepatitis D virus. In Mandell GL, Bennett JE, Dolin R, eds: *Principles and practices of infectious diseases,* ed 4, New York, 1995, Churchill Livingstone.
Schifman RB et al: Significance of isolated hepatitis B core antibody in blood donors, *Arch Intern Med* 153:2261-2266, 1993.

 What are the indications for HBV vaccination, serological evaluation following its administration, and booster dose?

*Indications for HBV vaccination:* all infants, preadolescents, adolescents, young adults, and persons with occupational risk or life-style risk (heterosexuals with multiple partners or any sexually transmitted disease, homosexual and bisexual men, injecting drug users, hemophiliac persons, hemodialysis patients, those having household and sexual contacts with hepatitis B virus carriers, clients and staff of institutions for the developmentally disabled, prisoners, immigrants and refugees from highly endemic areas, international travelers to HBV-endemic areas who will provide health care or will reside there more than 6 months or anticipate sexual contact with local persons).

*Indications for postvaccination serological testing:* persons whose subsequent clinical management depends on knowledge of their immune status (e.g., health care workers, hemodialysis patients, and infants born to HbsAg-positive mothers) and those with potential for suboptimal antibody response (e.g., 30 years or older, renal failure, HIV infection, diabetes, chronic liver disease, obesity, smoking, and vaccination in gluteus).

*Indications for booster dose:* none at this time (1997) for the majority of recipients (including health care workers) except for persons receiving hemodialysis in whom protection may decrease more rapidly; for these patients, annual serological testing should be performed and a booster HBV vaccine administered if antibody levels drop to less than 10 mIU/ml.

SUGGESTED READING

ACP Task Force on Adult Immunization and Infectious Diseases Society of America: Guide for adult immunization. Hepatitis B. In *Guide for adult immunization,* ed 3, Philadelphia, 1994, American College of Physicians.

## STIMULATING QUESTION

Should a child with chronic HBV carriage be allowed to enroll in school?

In the absence of behavioral problems (e.g., biting) or medical risk factors (e.g., generalized dermatitis or a bleeding problem), even in a day care setting, such children should be admitted to school without restriction.

SUGGESTED READING

Report of the Committee on Infectious Diseases: Hepatitis B. In Peter G, ed: *1997 Red Book: report of the Committee on Infectious Diseases,* ed 24, Elk Grove Village, Ill, 1997, American Academy of Pediatrics.

# Hepatitis C

 How should a positive hepatitis C virus (HCV) antibody in an asymptomatic person be interpreted?

Earlier seroepidemiological surveys indicated that up to 1.4% of sera of low-risk volunteer blood donors may be reactive by enzyme-linked immunoassays (EIAs). The first step is to determine if the seropositive person is truly infected with HCV. Only about 33% of initially seropositive volunteer blood donors by EIA, compared with 80% to 90% of EIA-positive parenteral drug users or transfusion recipients, will have positive results on supplemental ("confirmatory") testing.

The most widely used supplemental HCV antibody testing is the recombinant immunoblot assay (RIBA) test; a reactive supplemental test strongly supports a true-positive result and correlates well with detection of HCV genomic material in the blood by PCR. An indeterminate RIBA result, especially with second-generation RIBA, usually indicates nonspecific reactivity. However, because of the possibility of weak or indeterminate anti-HCV RIBA reactivity during the initial phase of HCV infection, follow-up serological testing may be necessary to exclude evolving antibody titers. Nevertheless, testing for HCV RNA by PCR should be strongly considered in patients with indeterminate anti-HCV RIBA; the presence of viral RNA in the blood of the donor supports viremia and HCV infection. Another viral detection test, quantitative bDNA signal amplification, is significantly less sensitive in detecting viremia than PCR test and should not be used to exclude HCV infection.

**120**

## ADDITIONAL POINTS TO REMEMBER

1. Most acute HCV infections are not clinically apparent; only 10% to 25% of patients with posttransfusion HCV infection become symptomatic.

2. About 75% of patients with HCV infection develop chronic hepatitis, of whom at least 20% develop cirrhosis, which may be complicated by hepatocellular carcinoma.

3. Mean interval between posttransfusion HCV infection and chronic hepatitis C, cirrhosis, and hepatocellular carcinoma is 10, 19, and 29 years, respectively.

4. Progression toward cirrhosis in HCV-infected individuals is probably facilitated by other risk factors such as concurrent hepatitis B or HIV infection and by hepatotoxic agents such as alcohol.

5. Alanine aminotransferase (ALT) levels in serum may be normal in 60% of individuals with HCV infection, with most (approximately 80%) having chronic persistent, occasionally chronic active, hepatitis with or without cirrhosis; therefore a normal ALT does not exclude the possibility of HCV infection.

### SUGGESTED READINGS

Becherer PR, Bacon B: Hepatitis C testing: interpretation, implications, and counseling, *Mo Med* 90:31-35, 1993.
Hsu HH et al: Antibodies to hepatitis C virus in low-risk blood donors: implications for counseling positive donors, *Gastroenterology* 101:1724-1727, 1991.
Scotiniotis I, Brass CA, Malet PF: Hepatitis C: diagnosis and treatment, *J Gen Intern Med* 10:273-282, 1995.
Tedeschi V, Seef LB: Diagnostic tests for hepatitis C: where are we now? *Ann Intern Med* 123:383-384, 1995 (editorial).
van der Poel CL, Cuypers HT, Reesink HW: Hepatitis C virus six years on, *Lancet* 344:1475-1479, 1994.

My patient was confirmed to be seropositive for HCV antibody. How should he or she be treated or managed?

Because of the frequently fluctuating nature of serum ALT in patients with HCV infection, this enzyme should be monitored periodically (i.e., every 6 months). Patients with persistently or intermittently elevated ALT and active inflammatory infiltrates on liver biopsy may benefit from interferon-alpha therapy (e.g., 3 million U subcutaneously 3×/wk for 6 months or longer). Proper therapy of individuals with normal serum ALT and less aggressive disease has not been defined.

*When considering interferon-alpha therapy,* the following factors should be considered:

1. It is not known whether interferon therapy will reduce the risk of major complications of HCV infection such as cirrhosis and liver cancer.

2. Chronic HCV infection is usually asymptomatic, whereas interferon therapy is often associated with significant side effects (e.g., flulike symptoms, leukopenia, thrombocytopenia, and psychiatric syndromes or depression), inconvenience of injections, and considerable expense.

3. In general, only 25% of treated patients can be expected to have a sustained response (i.e., normal ALT 6 months after cessation of therapy).

4. Long duration of HCV infection, older age, development of chronic active (rather than chronic persistent) hepatitis, cirrhosis, presence of HCV type Ib, or a high viral load at the start of treatment may be predictors of a less favorable response to interferon.

5. Decision to initiate therapy for any particular patient requires significant patient participation and subjective clinical judgment.

6. Whenever possible, referral of patients with HCV infection to research medical centers for participation in HCV treatment protocols is encouraged.

To date, studies of ribavirin, either alone or in combination with interferon-alpha in HCV infection, have generally shown disappointing results.

### SUGGESTED READINGS

Becherer PR, Bacon B: Hepatitis C testing: interpretation, implications, and counseling, *Mo Med* 90:31-35, 1993.

Lemon SM, Brown EA: Hepatitis C virus. In Mandell GL, Bennett JE, Dolin R, eds: *Principles and practices of infectious diseases,* ed 4, New York, 1995, Churchill Livingstone.

Scotiniotis I, Brass CA, Malet PF: Hepatitis C: diagnosis and treatment, *J Gen Intern Med* 10:273-282, 1995.

Scotto G et al: Treatment with ribavirin plus alpha interferon in HCV chronic active hepatitis non-responders to interferon alone: preliminary results, *J Chemother* 7:58-61, 1995.

van der Poel CL, Cuypers HT, Reesink HW: Hepatitis C virus six years on, *Lancet* 344:1475-1479, 1994.

 In addition to addressing treatment issues, how should patients with HCV infection be counseled?

Potential modes of transmission of HCV should be discussed with the patient. HCV is commonly found in blood, plasma, serum, and many other body fluids such as saliva, sweat, seminal fluid, breast milk, tears, and aqueous humor. Differentiation between HCV infection, other forms of hepatitis, and HIV should be stressed.

The classic risk factors for acquiring HCV include transfusion of blood or blood products, tissue or organ transplantation from infected donors, and IV drug abuse involving needle sharing. Other less commonly identified risk factors include tattoos placed under substandard conditions; contaminated needlestick injury in the health care setting (risk 1% to 10%); sexual contact with infected persons (risk 0% to 20%); casual household contact (less than 2% to 8%); and mother-infant transmission in utero, at delivery, or possibly during breast feeding (0% to 13%). No identifiable risk factors can be found in 44% of HCV-positive individuals. There is no evidence for transmission of HCV by insect bites or casual kissing.

Potential measures to reduce transmission of HCV should include the following:

1. Reduction in the number of sexual partners

2. Use of condoms, particularly outside mutually monogamous sexual behavior

3. Not sharing personal items such as toothbrushes, razors, manicure sets, or other items that may come in contact with blood; separate utensils and bathrooms are not necessary

4. Covering open skin lesions

5. HIV coinfected patients should be instructed that they may be at higher risk of transmitting HCV infection

6. Women of child-bearing age may place their offspring at risk (however low) of HCV infection by vertical transmission

Other points to stress to the patient include the following:

1. The clinical course of chronic hepatitis C infection in individual patients cannot be predicted

2. Patients should inform their health care providers of their HCV status

3. Potentially hepatotoxic insults such as alcohol (tenfold increase in risk of cirrhosis when concurrent with HCV infection) should be avoided

4. IV drug users should avoid sharing needles

5. HCV is not readily transmitted in the school settings or workplace; therefore no specific school or workplace restrictions are necessary

6. There is currently no proven-effective immunoglobulin preparation or vaccine for prevention of HCV pre- or post-exposure

7. Exposed sexual partners and household members should be considered for HCV testing

### SUGGESTED READINGS

Becherer PR, Bacon B: Hepatitis C testing: interpretation, implications, and counseling, *Mo Med* 90:31-35, 1993.

Caldwell SH et al: Sexual, vertical and household transmission of hepatitis C, *Virginia Med Q* 122:270-274, 1995.

Colquhoun SD: Hepatitis C: a clinical update, *Arch Surg* 131:18-23, 1996.

Lemon SM, Brown EA: Hepatitis C virus. In Mandell GL, Bennett JE, Dolin R, eds: *Principles and practices of infectious diseases*, ed 4, New York, 1995, Churchill Livingstone.

Seeff LB, Alter HJ: Spousal transmission of the hepatitis C virus, *Ann Intern Med* 120:807-809, 1994.

Seymour CA: Screening asymptomatic people at high risk for hepatitis C: the case for, *BMJ* 312:1347-1348, 1996.

Shapiro CN: Transmission of hepatitis viruses, *Ann Intern Med* 120:82-84, 1994.

A health care worker suffers a puncture injury by a contaminated needle from a patient who is HCV antibody positive. Is there a role for immunoglobulin prophylaxis?

The risk of transmission of HCV in this setting is 1% to 10%, depending on the study quoted. There is no recommended hyperimmune globulin or other treatment available for prophylaxis of HCV infection after a recognized exposure. Experimental studies in chimpanzees have not demonstrated efficacy of immunoglobulins in preventing HCV.

### SUGGESTED READINGS
Colquhoun SD: Hepatitis C: a clinical update, *Arch Surg* 131:18-23, 1996.
Krawczynski K et al: Effect of immune globulin on the prevention of experimental hepatitis C virus infection, *J Infect Dis* 173:822-828, 1996.
Sepkowitz KA: Occupationally acquired infections in health care workers. II, *Ann Intern Med* 125:917-928, 1996.

How should HCV infection in HIV-positive patients be managed? Is there a role for interferon-alpha treatment?

The natural course of chronic HCV infection in HIV-positive patients is largely unknown. In hemophiliac patients with concurrent HCV and HIV infection, liver failure may occur at a rate of 9% during the course of 10 to 20 years; however, the relative contribution of HCV (as compared with drugs or HIV) in this setting is unclear. In a study of predominantly non-IV drug-using HIV-infected male homosexuals, HCV infection did not appear to adversely influence survival of patients with or without AIDS. Studies of interferon-alpha therapy in limited number of patients with HIV and HCV infection with a mean CD4 lymphocyte count greater than 200 have shown similar response rates as those of HIV-negative patients. Whether treatment of HCV in patients with HIV infection will have any impact on overall survival or morbidity from HIV infection remains to be seen.

SUGGESTED READINGS

Boyer N et al: Recombinant interferon-alpha for chronic hepatitis C in patients positive for antibody to human immunodeficiency virus, *J Infect Dis* 165:723-726, 1992.

Eyster ME et al: Natural history of hepatitis C virus infection in multi-transfused hemophiliacs: effect of coinfection with human immunodeficiency virus, *J Acquir Immune Defic Syndr* 6:602-610, 1993.

Wright TL et al: Hepatitis C in HIV-infected patients with and without AIDS: prevalence and relationship to patient survival, *Hepatology* 20:1152-1155, 1994.

## STIMULATING QUESTION

Is it safe for a mother with HCV infection to breast feed her infant?

HCV has been found only rarely in breast milk. Whether positive specimens represent a risk of transmission to the infant is unclear but has been considered. Although there is no formal consensus on whether HCV-infected mothers may breast feed their infants, some investigators have suggested that this practice be allowed. The ultimate decision regarding this issue should be individualized, taking into account the potential benefits of breast feeding and thus far only theoretical risk of HCV transmission in this setting.

SUGGESTED READINGS

Caldwell SH et al: Sexual, vertical and household transmission of hepatitis C, *Virginia Med Q* 122:270-274, 1995.

Kurauchi O et al: Studies on transmission of hepatitis C virus from mother-to-child in the perinatal period, *Arch Gynecol Obstet* 253:121-126, 1993.

Ogasawara S et al: Hepatitis C virus RNA in saliva and breastmilk of hepatitis C carrier mothers, *Lancet* 341:561, 1993.

## STIMULATING QUESTION

Is it possible for someone to get reinfected with HCV? Does one develop immunity against future HCV infections?

Clinical studies involving liver transplant recipients and multitransfused hemophiliacs and experimental studies involving chimpanzees suggest that HCV infection does *not* elicit protective immunity against reinfection. Thus reinfection following exposure to heterologous strains of HCV is possible.

### SUGGESTED READINGS

Farci P et al: Lack of protective immunity against reinfection with hepatitis C virus, *Science* 258:135-140, 1992.

Feray C et al: Reinfection of liver graft by hepatitis C virus after liver transplantation, *J Clin Invest* 89:1361-1365, 1992.

Jarvis LM et al: Frequent reinfection and reactivation of hepatitis C virus genotypes in multitransfused hemophiliacs, *J Infect Dis* 170:1018-1022, 1994.

# Herpes Simplex Virus

 How is the diagnosis of herpes simplex virus (HSV) infection usually made?

Specimens from a variety of sites (e.g., cutaneous vesicles, oral ulcers, and respiratory secretions) may be cultured for herpes simplex using various tissue cell lines and looking for cytopathological effect within 24 to 48 hours of inoculation if the inoculum is high. Vesicles contain their highest viral titers within the first 24 to 48 hours of eruption. To improve the yield of cultures, specimens should be collected early during the course of disease and promptly inoculated into tissue cultures. Rapid diagnosis of possible herpes simplex infection may be made by scraping a lesion and staining with Giemsa preparation (Tzanck) smear, looking for multinucleated giant cells. However, a positive Tzanck smear cannot differentiate between herpes simplex and varicella virus infections.

Serological evaluation is of limited value in the diagnosis of recurrent infections. In primary infections, a fourfold or greater rise in antibody titers between acute and convalescent sera may be observed. The presence of IgM HSV antibodies in infants suggests recent infection. In older adults, IgM antibodies may not be useful in separating primary from recurrent infection.

HSV DNA detection in the cerebrospinal fluid by use of PCR is useful in the diagnosis of encephalitis caused by this virus. When compared with brain biopsy, it has a sensitivity of 98%,

**129**

specificity of 94%, positive predictive value of 95%, and negative predictive value of 98%, thus often obviating the need for brain biopsy.

## SUGGESTED READINGS

Hirsch MS: Herpes simplex virus. In Mandell GL, Bennett JE, Dolin R, eds: *Principles and practices of infectious diseases,* ed 4, New York, 1995, Churchill Livingstone.

Lakeman FD, Whitley RJ: Diagnosis of herpes simplex encephalitis: application of polymerase chain reaction to cerebrospinal fluid from brain-biopsied patients and correlation with disease, *J Infect Dis* 171:857-863, 1995.

 How should common herpes simplex infections in adults be managed or prevented?

## GENITAL INFECTION

Oral acyclovir (200 mg 5×/day for 10 days) or IV acyclovir (5 mg/kg every 8 hrs for 5 days) is the drug of choice for treatment of primary (initial attack) HSV genital infection; the latter is usually reserved for severe local infection or disease with systemic complications. Topical acyclovir (5% ointment every 6 hrs for 7 days) reduces the duration of viral shedding and the duration of time to crusting of the lesions, but it is not as effective as PO or IV therapy.

Recurrent genital herpes is usually less severe and resolves more rapidly than primary infection even without specific therapy. Topical acyclovir therapy has no significant effect on symptoms of patients with recurrent genital HSV infection. Oral acyclovir (200 mg 5×/day for 5 days) is usually recommended but has limited clinical benefit.

For long-term suppression of genital herpes in patients with frequent recurrences, oral acyclovir is recommended; the dose may be titrated down from 400 mg 2×/day to establish the minimal dose that is most effective in an individual patient. Therapy should be interrupted and reevaluated every 12 months to delineate continued need for suppression.

Note: *Although suppressive oral acyclovir (400 mg 2×/day) has been shown to significantly reduce (by 94%) asymptomatic shedding of HSV-2 in women with genital herpes of less than 2 years' duration, it is not clear whether acyclovir is effective in reducing sexual transmission of HSV. Therefore routine use of condoms and abstaining from sexual intercourse during recurrences are recommended.*

## HERPES LABIALIS (MUCOCUTANEOUS HSV IN IMMUNOCOMPETENT PATIENTS)

It is generally agreed that topical acyclovir has no appreciable clinical benefit on the course of herpes labialis ("fever blisters"), probably related to poor drug penetration. When initiated early during the prodromal or erythematous stages of infection, oral acyclovir (400 mg 5×/day for 5 days) may be of a slight clinical benefit by reducing the duration of pain by 36% and the length of time to the loss of crusts by 27%. Therefore routine treatment of herpes labialis is not recommended.

Oral acyclovir (400 mg 2×/day) is effective (53% reduction in the number of clinical recurrences) in suppressing herpes labialis in immunocompetent adults with recurrent infection and may be used short term to help prevent recurrence in patients who anticipate engaging in high-risk activities (e.g., intense and prolonged exposure to sunlight). Use of sunscreen preparations may also substantially reduce ultraviolet-light–induced herpes labialis in susceptible patients.

## ENCEPHALITIS

IV acyclovir 10 mg/kg every 8 hrs for 14 to 21 days is recommended. Treatment should be initiated without delay in suspected cases.

## INFECTION OF THE HAND (HERPETIC WHITLOW)

Oral acyclovir (200 mg 5×/day) for 10 days appears to significantly reduce pain and healing time. In frequently recurrent cases, prophylactic oral acyclovir (daily dose 600 to 1600 mg) may be effective.

Note: *The effectiveness of gloves in preventing transmission of HSV from health care personnel with herpetic whitlow is unknown. Therefore contact with patients during active infection is generally not recommended until the lesion(s) have healed. There is also no evidence that treatment of infected personnel with systemic acyclovir will eliminate the risk of transmission in this setting.*

### SUGGESTED READINGS

Gill MJ et al: Herpes simplex virus infection of the hand, *Am J Med* 85(suppl 2A):53-56, 1988.

Hirsch MS: Herpes simplex virus. In Mandell GL, Bennett JE, Dolin R, eds: *Principles and practices of infectious diseases,* ed 4, New York, 1995, Churchill Livingstone.

Rooney JF et al: Oral acyclovir to suppress frequently recurrent herpes labialis, *Ann Intern Med* 118:268-272, 1993.

Wald A et al: Suppression of subclinical shedding of herpes simplex virus type 2 with acyclovir, *Ann Intern Med* 124:8-15, 1996.

What isolation precautions are needed for the care of patients infected with HSV?

Standard precautions for avoidance of contact with potentially infected body fluids should be practiced. Specifically, direct contact with active lesions should be avoided, gloves should be worn when handling oral and vaginal secretions, and hands should be washed after patient contact.

### SUGGESTED READING

Adler SP: Herpes simplex. In Mandell GL, Bennett JE, Dolin R, eds: *Principles and practices of infectious diseases,* ed 4, New York, 1995, Churchill Livingstone.

Should a health care worker with herpetic whitlow, herpes labialis (fever blisters), or genital herpes be allowed to care for patients?

The effectiveness of gloves in preventing transmission of HSV from health care personnel with herpetic whitlow is unknown. Therefore contact with patients—particularly when immunocompromised (e.g., neonates, burn patients, and those with immunodeficiencies or severe malnutrition) or in the intensive care unit—during active infection is generally not recommended until the lesion(s) have healed. There is also no evidence that treatment of infected personnel with systemic acyclovir will eliminate the risk of transmission in this setting. Strict observance of hand washing is essential in minimizing the risk of transmission.

Personnel with active herpes labialis generally should not care for immunocompromised patients (see above) unless their services are absolutely essential, in which case the following precautions should be taken: (1) cover and avoid touching the lesions; (2) observe strict hand washing techniques; and (3) avoid kissing or nuzzling patients (e.g., newborn infants or children with dermatitis).

There is no evidence that health care workers with genital herpes infection pose a high risk to patients, as long as they follow good patient care practices (e.g., hand washing). Therefore such personnel are usually allowed to care for patients.

SUGGESTED READINGS

Adler SP: Herpes simplex. In Mayhall CG, ed: *Hospital epidemiology and infection control,* Baltimore, 1996, Williams & Wilkins.
American Academy of Pediatrics: Herpes simplex. In Peter G, ed: *1997 Red Book: report of the Committee on Infectious Diseases,* ed 24, Elk Grove Village, Ill, 1997, American Academy of Pediatrics.

## STIMULATING QUESTION

When is it safe to kiss someone with history of recurrent herpes labialis (fever blisters)?

Recurrent herpes labialis involving the lips or perioral area occurs in 20% to 40% of the population and is usually caused by herpes simplex virus type 1. Viral shedding, and most likely infectiveness, is highest during the first 24 hours or vesicular stage, with significant decline in viral titers thereafter, such that after 5 days when most lesions have healed viral recovery is unlikely. However, because as many as 24% of adults may asymptomatically shed herpes simplex in their saliva, it would be reasonable to assume that kissing a person with history of recurrent herpes labialis will be "safer" after complete healing of the lesion but that the risk will not necessarily be zero even in the absence of an active lesion.

## SUGGESTED READINGS

Spruance SL et al: The natural history of recurrent herpes simplex labialis: implications for antiviral therapy, *N Engl J Med* 297:69-75, 1977.
Turner R et al: Shedding and survival of herpes simplex virus from "fever blisters," *Pediatrics* 70:547-549, 1982.

## STIMULATING QUESTION

Are spermicides effective in preventing transmission of genital herpes?

Although spermicides such as nonoxynol-9 when used in conjunction with condoms have been associated with reduction in rate of gonococcal and chlamydial cervical infections, their efficacy in prevention of herpes infections has not been clinically studied. However, nonoxynol-9 and nonoxynol-11 have been shown to inhibit herpes simplex virus type 2 and HIV in vitro.

## SUGGESTED READINGS

Jennings R, Clegg A: The inhibitory effect of spermicidal agents on replication of HSV-2 and HIV-1 in-vitro, *J Antimicrob Chemother* 32:71-82, 1993.
Niruthisard S, Roddy RE, Chutivongse S: Use of nonoxynol-9 and reduction in rate of gonococcal and chlamydial cervical infections, *Lancet* 339:1371-1375, 1992.

# Herpes Zoster

 How should herpes zoster (shingles) be treated?

## IMMUNOCOMPETENT PATIENTS

Acyclovir 800 mg 5×/day PO for 7 days, started within 72 hrs of rash, has been shown to significantly reduce the time to last new lesion formation, loss of vesicles, and full crusting, without effects on the frequency or severity of postherpetic neuralgia. In "relatively healthy" persons (e.g., immunocompetent patients or those without cancer, hypertension, osteoporosis, glycosuria, or diabetes), use of acyclovir 800 mg 5×/day PO for 21 days with prednisone (60 mg for the first week, 30 mg/day for the second week, and 15 mg/day for the third week) may improve quality of life (acute neuritis pain and return to uninterrupted sleep and usual daily activity) but not postherpetic neuralgia.

In patients 50 years old or older, valaciclovir 1000 mg 3×/day for 7 days (begun within 72 hrs of rash) may be superior to acyclovir 800 mg 5×/day for 7 days in significantly accelerating the resolution of herpes zoster–associated pain and reducing the duration of postherpetic neuralgia.

Famciclovir 500 mg 3×/day (started within 72 hrs of rash) has also been shown to accelerate healing of cutaneous lesions and reduce postherpetic neuralgia (median by 2 months).

**136**

## IMMUNOCOMPROMISED HOSTS

See section under "Immunocompromised Host."

### SUGGESTED READINGS

Beutner KR et al: Valaciclovir compared with acyclovir for improved therapy for herpes zoster in immunocompetent adults, *Antimicrob Agents Chemother* 39:1546-1553, 1995.

Tyring S et al: Famciclovir for the treatment of acute herpes zoster: effects on acute disease and postherpetic neuralgia, *Ann Intern Med* 123:89-96, 1995.

Whitley RJ, Gnann JW: Acyclovir: a decade later, *N Engl J Med* 327:782-789, 1992.

Whitley RJ et al: Acyclovir with and without prednisone for the treatment of herpes zoster. A randomized, placebo-controlled trial, *Ann Intern Med* 125:376-383, 1996.

 What isolation precautions should be followed when caring for hospitalized patients with herpes zoster?

Varicella-zoster virus (VZV) can be transmitted from the lesions of patients who have herpes zoster to susceptible contacts, resulting in primary varicella in these persons. However, the likelihood of transmission of VZV is much less than from primary varicella.

Immunocompetent patients with herpes zoster should be placed on contact precautions to prevent transmission by direct or indirect contact with infectious material/drainage from actively infected lesions. Visitors and staff with no history of chicken pox should not enter the room unless proof of immunity can be obtained by serological testing. The patient is considered infectious until the drainage from lesions has ceased.

Immunocompromised patients with herpes zoster should be placed in a private room with negative air pressure relative to the corridor whenever possible. Persons without history of chicken pox should not enter the room. Strict isolation including use of mask, gown, and gloves when entering the room should be observed for all persons until all skin lesions have crusted.

## SUGGESTED READINGS

Centers for Disease Control and Prevention: Prevention of varicella. Recommendations of the advisory committee on immunization practices (ACIP), *MMWR* 45(RR-11):1-36, 1996.

Garner JS: Guidelines for isolation precautions in hospitals, *Infect Control Hosp Epidemiol* 17:53-80, 1996.

Zaia JA: Varicella-zoster virus. In Mayhall CG, ed: *Hospital epidemiology and infection control,* Baltimore, 1996, Williams & Wilkins.

 Can VZV reactivate and cause herpes zoster–like symptoms without associated cutaneous eruption? If so, how can this condition be diagnosed?

*Zoster sine herpete* is the term used to describe segmental pain without cutaneous eruption as a result of reactivation of varicella-zoster in the dorsal root ganglion. Serological evidence of seroconversion or significant increase in antibodies (e.g., fluorescence antibody to membrane antigen [FAMA] or enzyme-linked immunosorbent assays [ELISAs]) against VZV supports the diagnosis.

## SUGGESTED READINGS

Arvin AM: Immune responses to varicella-zoster virus, *Infect Dis Clin North Am* 10:529-570, 1996.

Gilden DH et al: Varicella-zoster reactivation without rash, *J Infect Dis* 166(suppl 1):S30-S34, 1992.

Mayo DR, Booss J: Varicella zoster–associated neurologic disease without skin lesions, *Arch Neurol* 48:313-315, 1989.

Whitley RJ: Varicella-zoster virus. In Mandell GL, Bennett JE, Dolin R, eds: *Principles and practices of infectious diseases,* ed 4, New York, 1995, Churchill Livingstone.

## STIMULATING QUESTION

Can cerebrospinal fluid pleocytosis occur as a result of herpes zoster?

Elevated cerebrospinal white blood cell counts have been associated with herpes zoster, as well as zoster without cutaneous eruption.

### SUGGESTED READINGS

Mayo DR, Booss J: Varicella zoster–associated neurologic disease without skin lesions, *Arch Neurol* 48:313-315, 1989.
Whitley RJ: Varicella-zoster virus. In Mandell GL, Bennett JE, Dolin R, eds: *Principles and practices of infectious diseases,* ed 4, New York, 1995, Churchill Livingstone.

## STIMULATING QUESTION

Should a surgeon with herpes zoster be allowed to perform surgery?

Immunocompetent health care workers with localized herpes zoster may be allowed to work as long as their cutaneous lesions can be adequately covered and their contacts are not immunocompromised and are considered immune to varicella.

### SUGGESTED READING

Zaia JA: Varicella-zoster virus. In Mayhall CG, ed: *Hospital epidemiology and infection control,* Baltimore, 1996, Williams & Wilkins.

# Human Immunodeficiency Virus

 How should health care workers be managed after exposure involving HIV-contaminated needles?

## GENERAL ISSUES

Health care workers exposed to HIV should receive appropriate counseling and serological testing for HIV antibody (usually by ELISA) as soon as possible after exposure. A negative baseline HIV antibody test should help establish occupation-related nature of the infection if seroconversion occurs during the ensuing 6 months (rate 0.3%). HIV antibody testing should be considered at 6 weeks, 3 months, and 6 months after exposure. Testing beyond 6 months should not be routinely performed because of unlikelihood of seroconversion after this period and the prolongation of health care workers' anxiety regarding possible transmission of HIV. Exposed persons should also return for evaluation if symptoms or signs associated with acute retroviral infection (e.g., unexplained fever, lymphadenopathy, rash, pharyngitis, or aseptic meningitis) develop. In some cases, supportive counseling by trained clinicians and professionals may be necessary to help the exposed person cope with the stress and anxiety associated with such exposure. The exposed health care worker should also be advised to avoid exchange of body fluids during sexual contact and to defer pregnancy, breast feeding, and blood and organ donation during the 6-month follow-up.

## CHEMOPROPHYLAXIS

Chemoprophylaxis with zidovudine (AZT) has been associated with a decrease of 79% in the risk for HIV seroconversion after percutaneous exposure to HIV-infected blood. Based on this finding, the Centers for Disease Control and Prevention have recommended the chemoprophylactic regimen below for health care workers with occupational exposure to HIV (Table 1). Chemoprophylaxis should be initiated promptly, preferably within 1 to 2 hours postexposure; the interval beyond which prophylaxis may be ineffective is unknown. Even if infection is not prevented, early treatment of acute HIV infection may be beneficial.

Drug toxicity should be monitored by obtaining a blood count and renal and hepatic chemical tests at baseline and 2 weeks after start of chemoprophylaxis. If subjective or objective toxicity is noted, dose reduction or drug substitution should be considered with the assistance of an expert in HIV infection.

### SUGGESTED READINGS

Centers for Disease Control and Prevention: Public Health Service statement on management of occupational exposure to human immunodeficiency virus, including considerations regarding zidovudine postexposure use, *MMWR* 39(RR-1):1-14, 1990.

Centers for Disease Control and Prevention: Update: provisional public health service recommendations for chemoprophylaxis after occupational exposure to HIV, *MMWR* 45:468-472, 1996.

Gerberding JL: Management of occupational exposure to blood-borne viruses, *N Engl J Med* 332:444-451, 1995.

Gerberding JL, Henderson DK: Management of occupational exposures to bloodborne pathogens: hepatitis B virus, hepatitis C virus, and human immunodeficiency virus, *Clin Infect Dis* 14:1179-1185, 1992.

TABLE 1 *Provisional Public Health Service recommendations for chemoprophylaxis after occupational exposure to HIV, by type of exposure and source material—1996*

| Type of Exposure | Source Material[a] | Antiretroviral Prophylaxis[b] | Antiretroviral Regimen[c] |
|---|---|---|---|
| Percutaneous | Blood[d] | | |
| | Highest risk | Recommend | ZDV, 3TC, and IDV |
| | Increased risk | Recommend | ZDV and 3TC, ± IDV[e] |
| | No increased risk | Offer | ZVD and 3TC |
| | Fluid containing visible blood, other potentially infectious fluid,[f] or tissue | Offer | ZDV and 3TC |
| | Other body fluid (e.g., urine) | Not offer | |
| Mucous membranes | Blood | Offer | ZDV and 3TC, ± IDV[e] |
| | Fluid containing visible blood, other potentially infectious fluid,[f] or tissue | Offer | ZDV, ± 3TC |
| | Other body fluid (e.g., urine) | Not offer | |
| Skin, increased risk[g] | Blood | Offer | ZDV and 3TC, ± IDV[e] |
| | Fluid containing visible blood, other potentially infectious fluid,[f] or tissue | Offer | ZDV, ± 3TC |
| | Other body fluid (e.g., urine) | Not offer | |

[a] Any exposure to concentrated HIV (e.g., in a research laboratory or production facility) is treated as percutaneous exposure to blood with highest risk.

[b] *Recommend,* Postexposure prophylaxis should be recommended to the exposed worker with counseling. *Offer,* Postexposure prophylaxis should be offered to the exposed worker with counseling. *Not offer,* Postexposure prophylaxis should not be offered because these are not occupational exposures to HIV.

[c] Regimens: Zidovudine (ZDV), 200 mg 3×/day; lamivudine (3TC), 150 mg 2×/day; indinavir (IDV), 800 mg 3×/day (if IDV is not available, saquinavir may be used, 600 mg 3×/day). Prophylaxis is given for 4 weeks. For full prescribing information, see package inserts.

[d] *Highest risk,* BOTH larger volume of blood (e.g., deep injury with large-diameter hollow needle previously in source patient's vein or artery, especially involving an injection of source patient's blood) AND blood containing a high titer of HIV (e.g., source with acute retroviral illness or end-stage AIDS; viral load measurement may be considered, but its use in relation to postexposure prophylaxis has not been evaluated). *Increased risk,* EITHER exposure to larger volume of blood OR blood with a high titer of HIV. *No increased risk,* NEITHER exposure to larger volume of blood NOR blood with a high titer of HIV (e.g., solid suture needle injury from source patient with asymptomatic HIV infection).

[e] Possible toxicity of additional drug may not be warranted.

[f] Includes semen; vaginal secretions; and cerebrospinal, synovial, pleural, peritoneal, pericardial, and amniotic fluids.

[g] For skin, risk is increased for exposures involving a high titer of HIV, prolonged contact, an extensive area, or an area in which skin integrity is visibly compromised. For skin exposures without increased risk, the risk for drug toxicity outweighs the benefit of postexposure prophylaxis.

What is the risk of HIV transmission in various situations and populations?

Sexual intercourse: Heterosexual (approximately 0.1%); in Thailand female-to-male, 5.6% (average per contact). Male-to-male, approximately 1%. Efficiency of transmission may be higher from male-to-female than female-to-male.

Injection drug use: Seroconversion varies from 1% to 60% depending on city (New York City 34% to 61%; New Orleans 1%).

Blood transfusions: Estimated 1 in 230,000 per unit of blood following implementation of routine HIV testing of all donors.

Hemophiliacs: Incidence decreased significantly following routine HIV testing of all donors (17 new cases from April, 1985 through 1988).

Perinatal transmission: 25% to 40% of infants born of seropositive mothers may be infected. Zidovudine can reduce risk to 8%.

Occupational exposure: 0.3% to 0.4% for percutaneous exposures; risks for other types of exposures probably lower.

Home care providers: None of over 1100 persons living with HIV-infected patients tested showed evidence of household transmission.

Note: *Transmission rates vary depending on host-related factors (susceptibility and infectiousness), environmental factors (social, cultural), and agent factors (HIV type I). Host infectiousness is likely to increase as the concentration of virus in the blood or genital tract increases, as is often observed in patients with low CD4 lymphocyte counts and advanced HIV disease.*

SUGGESTED READINGS

Bartlett JG: Estimates and mechanisms of transmission of human immunodeficiency virus in the United States, *Infect Dis Clin Pract* 3:173-174, 1994.

Connor EM et al: Reduction of maternal-infant transmission of human immunodeficiency virus type I with zidovudine treatment, *N Engl J Med* 331:1173-1180, 1994.

MacDonald MG, Ginzburg HM, Bolan JC: HIV infection in pregnancy: epidemiology and clinical management, *J AIDS* 4:100-108, 1991.

Royce RA, Sena A, Cates W: Sexual transmission of HIV, *N Engl J Med* 336:1072-1078, 1997.

 When should antiretroviral therapy be considered in adults with HIV infection?

Antiretroviral therapy is recommended for all patients with symptomatic HIV disease (including AIDS, weight loss, chronic unexplained fever, oral hairy leukoplakia, and recurrent mucosal candidiasis). For asymptomatic patients with CD4+ count <500/µl, therapy is generally recommended; some experts would defer therapy in patients with stable CD4+ cell counts between 350 and 500/µl and plasma HIV RNA levels consistently below 5000 to 10,000 copies/ml. Therapy is also recommended for patients with greater than 30,000 to 50,000 HIV RNA copies/ml or rapidly declining CD4+ cell counts (greater than 300 loss over 12 to 18 months) and should be considered for patients with greater than 5000 to 10,000 HIV RNA copies/ml.

Note: *There are no clinical data to support treatment of HIV infection in patients with CD4+ >500. In this subset of patients, decision regarding treatment should also take into account the potential long-term toxicity, expense, tolerance, and possible induction of drug resistance.*

Choice of initial therapy: zidovudine (AZT) and didanosine (ddl), or zidovudine and zalcitabine (ddC), or zidovudine and lamivudine (3TC), or didanosine monotherapy.

Other possible candidates for initial therapy (formal clinical studies unavailable): stavudine (D4T) and didanosine, and stavudine and 3TC. *Avoid zalcitabine, zidovudine, and lamivudine monotherapy.*

It may be reasonable to include a protease inhibitor in the initial regimen for symptomatic patients, those with lower or rapidly decreasing CD4 cell counts, and those with high plasma HIV RNA levels. Selection of a protease inhibitor (e.g., saquinavir, ritonavir, and indinavir) should be based on its efficacy, potency, safety, tolerability, durability of antiviral effects, drug resistance patterns, potential for limiting future treatment options, and cost.

SUGGESTED READING

Carpenter CC et al: Antiretroviral therapy for HIV infection in 1996, *JAMA* 276:146-154, 1996.

 How long does it take for antibodies to HIV to develop following acute infection?

The majority (95%) of seroconversions occur within 6 months of exposure. To date all health care workers with known occupational exposure to HIV have seroconverted within 6 months and most within 4 months of exposure.

Note: *Often there is a confusion between time to seroconversion and time to development of AIDS. It usually takes only a few months to determine if someone has developed HIV infection following an exposure by detection of HIV antibody in the serum. However, it may take years (often 8 to 10 years or longer) before AIDS develops in an HIV-infected patient.*

SUGGESTED READINGS

Henderson DK: HIV in the healthcare setting. In Mandell GL, Bennett JE, Dolin R, eds: *Principles and practices of infectious diseases*, ed 4, New York, 1995, Churchill Livingstone.

Horburgh C et al: Duration of human immunodeficiency virus infection before detection of antibody, *Lancet* 2:637-640, 1989.

What infection control guidelines are recommended for the care of patients with HIV infection in health care settings?

There are usually no special precautions for the care of HIV patients. Blood and body fluids of *all* patients should be considered potentially infectious, and therefore direct exposure to such substances should be avoided (universal precautions or body substance isolation). Gloves, gowns, goggles, and masks should be worn as appropriate whenever blood or body fluid exposure is anticipated. Needlesticks should be avoided. Standard sterilization and disinfection procedures for patient care equipment are considered adequate for items contaminated with body fluids of patients with HIV infection. Extraordinary attempts to disinfect or sterilize environmental surfaces (e.g., walls and floors) are not necessary. All spills of blood and blood-contaminated fluids should be promptly cleaned by gloved hands with an appropriate Environmental Protection Agency–approved disinfectant or a 1:100 solution of household bleach.

SUGGESTED READING

Bell DM, Curran JW: Human immunodeficiency virus infection. In Bennett JV, Brachman PS, eds: *Hospital infections*, Boston, 1992, Little, Brown.

## STIMULATING QUESTION

Does mononucleosis cause HIV seropositivity?

Acute DNA viral infections have been reported to be associated with false-positive HIV antibody by ELISA in 5% of cases. False-positive HIV antibody detected by certain ELISA assays has been reported in association with positive heterophile antibody (Paul-Bunnell). Although false-positive HIV antibody may be observed in the setting of acute mononucleosis, the confirmatory test (e.g., Western blot) should remain nonreactive.

### SUGGESTED READINGS

Mortimer PP, Parry JV, Mortimer JY: Which anti-HTLVIII/LAV assays for screening and confirmatory testing? *Lancet* 2:873-877, 1985.

Steckelberg JM, Cockerill FR III: Serologic testing for human immunodeficiency virus antibodies, *Mayo Clin Proc* 63:373-380, 1988.

# Human Parvovirus B19

Q  What are the common clinical manifestations of
acute human parvovirus B19 (HPV-B19) infection?

Acute HPV-B19 infection may be subclinical or associated
with symptoms and a biphasic illness. Within a week after
infection, viremia causes a brief, mild nonspecific illness
consisting of fever, malaise, myalgias, headache, and pruritus. The more characteristic sign of HPV-B19 infection—
erythema infectiosum, or fifth disease (named as the "fifth"
of the originally described childhood exanthematous diseases)—develops approximately 10 days later, during the
"immune phase" of the illness when viremia can no longer
be detected. Fifth disease is more common in children and
is associated with a slapped cheek appearance sparing the
circumoral region; a lacy pink rash may also occur on the
extremities and on the trunk. The rash often resolves
within a week but may recur episodically for several weeks
from exposure to heat (e.g., during bathing), cold, exercise,
or stress.

In adults, arthralgia and arthritis are observed more commonly (as high as 60%), particularly in women, during the
"immune phase" of the disease. Symmetrical peripheral polyarthropathy involving particularly the joints of the hands,
wrists, and knees is common. Although the joint symptoms
are usually self-limited, they may last months to years.
Chronic arthritis is rare.

Anemia, thrombocytopenia, and leukopenia may develop in normal hosts with acute HPV-B19 infection but are usually asymptomatic and last about a week. In patients with chronic hemolytic anemias such as in sickle-cell anemia or with hereditary spherocytosis, malaria, and thalassemia, a transient aplastic crisis with severe anemia may occur. Accelerated hematopoiesis as a result of shortened red blood cell survival provides optimal medullary conditions for the growth of HPV-B19.

HPV-B19 may mimic or exacerbate systemic lupus erythematosus (SLE). Vasculitis, polyarteritis nodosa, and Henoch-Schönlein purpura have also been reported.

Acute HPV-B19 infection during pregnancy presents similar to the infection in other adults but can result in nonimmune fetal hydrops in a minority of cases (see the following section).

## SUGGESTED READINGS

Naides SJ et al: Rheumatologic manifestations of human parvovirus B19 infection in adults. Initial two-year clinical experience, *Arthritis Rheum* 33:1297-1309, 1990.

Nesher G, Osborn TG, Moore TL: Parvovirus infection mimicking systemic lupus erythematosus, *Semin Arthritis Rheum* 24:297-303, 1995.

Portmore AC: Parvoviruses (erythema infectiosum, aplastic crisis). In Mandell GL, Bennett JE, Dolin R, eds: *Principles and practices of infectious diseases,* ed 4, New York, 1995, Churchill Livingstone.

Rotbart HA: Human parvovirus infections, *Ann Rev Med* 41:25-34, 1990.

 How is acute parvovirus B19 infection diagnosed?

The principle means of diagnosis of acute parvovirus B19 infection in adults is by detection of viral-specific IgM antibody by EIA; it has a sensitivity of 97% in patients with erythema infectiosum (fifth disease) and a specificity of 96%. Anti–parvovirus HPV-B19 IgM may be present as early as 3 days after onset of symptoms of viremia and can persist for up to 6 months, sometimes longer. IgG antibodies against parvovirus HPV-B19 develop several days after IgM detection and persists for years, probably for life. PCR on blood or other body fluids may be used to determine the presence of parvovirus viremia, particularly when serological testing is not helpful and active viremia is suspected (e.g., immunocompromised patients).

In the presence of erythema infectiosum, the classic clinical features (slapped cheek appearance sparing the circumoral region), particularly in a child, are often sufficient for the diagnosis.

### SUGGESTED READINGS

Erdman DD et al: Human parvovirus B19 specific IgG, IgA, and IgM antibodies and DNA in serum specimens from persons with erythema infectiosum, *J Med Virol* 35:110-115, 1991.

Morinet F et al: Development of an IgM antibody capture test using labeled fusion protein as antigen for diagnosis of B19 human parvovirus infections, *Behring Inst Mitt* (Aug):28-34, 1990.

Portmore AC: Parvoviruses (erythema infectiosum, aplastic crisis). In Mandell GL, Bennett JE, Dolin R, eds: *Principles and practices of infectious diseases,* ed 4, New York, 1995, Churchill Livingstone.

Schwarz TF et al: Diagnosis of human parvovirus B19 infections by polymerase chain reaction, *Scand J Infect Dis* 24:691-696, 1992.

 How is HPV-B19 transmitted?

Parvovirus B19 is presumed to be transmitted primarily by respiratory secretions. The virus can be transmitted after exposure by close person-to-person contact in household, school, and day care settings. Nosocomial and laboratory transmission may also occur.

This virus may also be transmitted parenterally from contaminated blood products: single-donor blood products, risk 1:50,000; much higher risk for clotting factor concentrates. Tattoos have also been suspected as a mode of transmission. Vertical transmission from mother to fetus has also been well documented and can be associated with hydrops fetalis. Humans are the only known hosts for HPV-B19.

## SUGGESTED READING

Portmore AC: Parvoviruses (erythema infectiosum, aplastic crisis). In Mandell GL, Bennett JE, Dolin R, eds: *Principles and practices of infectious diseases*, ed 4, New York, 1995, Churchill Livingstone.

 What is the risk of transmission of parvovirus to a pregnant health care worker, and how should she be counseled after caring for an infected patient?

The risk of parvovirus transmission to a susceptible health care worker exposed to children with chronic hemolytic anemias and aplastic crisis (a condition associated with B19 infection) may be as high as 38%. Because immunity following parvovirus infection is thought to be lifelong, the presence of viral-specific IgG antibody in the absence of IgM antibody in the exposed person suggests probable immunity. In contrast, in the absence of detectable viral-specific IgG antibody, the exposed pregnant health care worker should be considered susceptible and should be counseled accordingly.

Exposed women who are both IgG and IgM negative for specific antibodies initially are at risk of infection and should be retested in 3 weeks. Evidence of IgM positivity supports the diagnosis of acute HPV-B19 infection, although false-positive IgM may also occur.

Pregnancy does not adversely affect the course of infection, but infection may have an adverse effect on the course of pregnancy. Although HPV-B19 can be transmitted vertically from mother to fetus (rate approximately 30%), the risk of an associated adverse fetal outcome (e.g., hydrops fetalis) in this setting has been estimated to be less than 10%. An excessive frequency of fetal loss during the second trimester has been observed. Infants who survive HPV-B19 infection have been reported to be normal at 1 year of age. Therefore therapeutic abortion of the infected fetus is not recommended.

Aside from the risk of fetal infection, the susceptible exposed adult should be advised of the possibility of developing symptomatic parvovirus disease such as arthritis and, less frequently, erythema infectiosum and vasculitis. The incubation period is 1 to 2 weeks.

There are no studies on whether pre- or postexposure prophylaxis with immunoglobulin modifies the course of illness or prevents infection; therefore routine prophylaxis cannot be recommended at this time.

### SUGGESTED READINGS

Alger LS: Toxoplasmosis and parvovirus B19, *Infect Dis Clin North Am* 11:55-75, 1997.

Gillespie SM et al: Occupational risk of human parvovirus B19 infection for school and day-care personnel during an outbreak of erythema infectiosum, *JAMA* 263:2061-2065, 1990.

Portmore AC: Parvoviruses (erythema infectiosum, aplastic crisis). In Mandell GL, Bennett JE, Dolin R, eds: *Principles and practices of infectious diseases,* ed 4, New York, 1995, Churchill Livingstone.

Public Health Laboratory Service Working Party on Fifth Disease: Prospective study of human parvovirus (B19) infection in pregnancy, *BMJ* 300:1166-1170, 1990.

Rotbart HA: Human parvovirus infections, *Ann Rev Med* 41:25-34, 1990.

# Human T-Lymphotropic Virus Type I and Type II

Q What is the significance of a positive human T-cell lymphotropic virus (HTLV) types I and II antibody in an asymptomatic person?

A blood specimen that is repeatedly reactive for HTLV-I and -II antibody by enzyme immunoassay and confirmed reactive by more specific tests such as Western immunoblot or radioimmunoprecipitation assay is considered positive. Differentiation of HTLV-I and -II antibodies is not usually possible with the use of the commonly available tests. The seroprevalence rate of HTLV-I and -II antibodies among volunteer blood donors is 0.016%.

HTLV-I infection is endemic in southwestern Japan, the Caribbean basin, Melanesia, and parts of Africa. Clusters of HTLV-I infections have also been reported among blacks living in the southeastern United States and in immigrants from endemic countries living in Brooklyn, New York. HTLV-I has been associated with adult T-cell leukemia/lymphoma (ATL) and myelopathy and tropical spastic paraparesis. The risk of ATL is 2% to 4%, often occurring several decades after infection.

HTLV-I–associated myelopathy/tropical spastic paraparesis is characterized by progressive and permanent weakness of the lower extremities, spasticity, hyperreflexia, sensory disturbances, and urinary incontinence and occurs in less than 1% of those infected with this virus.

**153**

HTLV-II is endemic in American Indian populations and is prevalent among injecting drug users in the United States. Infection caused by this virus has not been clearly associated with any diseases, although rare cases of myelopathy and tropical spastic paraparesis-like neurological illnesses, mycosis fungoides, and large granular lymphocyte leukemia have been reported in those infected.

It is worth stressing that the majority (more than 95%) of patients testing positive for HTLV-I and -II antibodies will remain asymptomatic from this infection. Nevertheless, periodic follow-up of HTLV-I infected persons by a physician knowledgeable about this virus is recommended. Physical examination, including a complete neurological examination and a complete blood count with peripheral smear examination are suggested. Medical evaluation of HTLV-II–infected persons is considered optional at this time.

### SUGGESTED READING

Centers for Disease Control and Prevention and the USPHS Working Group: Guidelines for counseling persons infected with human T-lymphotropic virus type I (HTLV-I) and type II (HTLV-II), *Ann Intern Med* 118:448-454, 1993.

 How are HTLV-I and -II transmitted?

HTLV-I may be transmitted by blood transfusion, sexual contact, sharing of contaminated needles, and from mother to child, primarily through breast feeding; intrauterine or perinatal transmission is less frequent. Mode of transmission of HTLV-II is less well characterized but is thought to be similar to that of HTLV-I.

## SUGGESTED READING

Centers for Disease Control and Prevention and the USPHS Working Group: Guidelines for counseling persons infected with human T-lymphotropic virus type I (HTLV-I) and type II (HTLV-II), *Ann Intern Med* 118:448-454, 1993.

 How should asymptomatic HTLV-I and -II seropositive persons be counseled?

General information regarding these viruses, the lifelong nature of infections associated with them, their probability of association with certain diseases, and their modes of transmission should be thoroughly discussed with the patient. The patient should inform his or her physician(s) of seropositive results. It should be stressed to the patient that HTLV-I and -II are not associated with AIDS.

The following advice should also be given to reduce the risk of transmission of these viruses:

1. Do not donate blood, semen, body organs, or other tissues.
2. Do not breast feed infants.
3. Do not share needles or syringes with others.
4. Consider the use of latex condoms to prevent sexual transmission.
5. If the seropositive individual is in a mutually monogamous sexual relationship, the partner should be tested also to help formulate specific counseling advice.
   a. If the partner is seropositive, no further recommendations are indicated.
   b. If the partner is seronegative, use of latex condoms is advised. Male-infected, female-noninfected couples de-

siring pregnancy should be made aware of a small risk for sexual transmission of HTLV-I during attempts at pregnancy, as well as finite risk for vertical transmission from mother to infant independent of breast feeding.

6. Infected persons with multiple sex partners or otherwise engaging in non–mutually monogamous sexual relationships should use latex condoms.

SUGGESTED READING

Centers for Disease Control and Prevention and the USPHS Working Group: Guidelines for counseling persons infected with human T-lymphotropic virus type I (HTLV-I) and type II (HTLV-II), *Ann Intern Med* 118:448-454, 1993.

How should persons with "indeterminate" HTLV-I and -II antibody tests be managed?

Persons testing "indeterminate" should be retested at least 3 months following the original test. If the repeat test is also "indeterminate," they should be reassured that they are not likely to be infected with HTLV-I or -II virus.

SUGGESTED READING

Centers for Disease Control and Prevention and the USPHS Working Group: Guidelines for counseling persons infected with human T-lymphotropic virus type I (HTLV-I) and type II (HTLV-II), *Ann Intern Med* 118:448-454, 1993.

# Imipenem

Q   What are the risk factors for imipenem/cilastatin (Primaxin)–induced seizures?

Seizures occur in 1% to 3% of patients treated with imipenem and are associated with lesions of the CNS, history of seizure activity, renal insufficiency, and excessive doses. Simultaneous use of imipenem/cilastatin with theophylline or cyclosporin may increase the risk of seizures.

To minimize the risk of seizures, standard dosages of imipenem for adults should be kept at or below 2 g or 25 mg/kg/day, whichever is less, unless dictated by specific clinical or microbiological circumstances. Furthermore, imipenem should be avoided in patients with bacterial meningitis because of its epileptogenic properties.

## SUGGESTED READINGS

Bosmuller C et al: Increased risk of central nervous system toxicity in patients treated with cyclosporin and imipenem/cilastatin, *Nephron* 58:362-364, 1991.

Hellinger WC, Brewer NS: Imipenem, *Mayo Clin Proc* 66:1074-1081, 1991.

Manian FA, Stone WJ, Alford RH: Adverse antibiotic effects associated with renal insufficiency, *Rev Infect Dis* 12:236-249, 1990.

Semel JD, Allen N: Seizures in patients simultaneously receiving theophylline and imipenem or ciprofloxacin or metronidazole, *South Med J* 84:465-468, 1991.

How should the dose of IV imipenem/cilastatin (Primaxin) be adjusted in renal insufficiency?

For adult patients with glomerular filtration rate (GFR) greater than 30 ml/min/1.73 m$^2$, the standard dose of 500 mg every 6 to 8 hrs is recommended. For patients with GFR of 10 to 30 ml/min/1.73 m$^2$, the daily dose should be 50% of that for patients with normal renal function and the same clinical and microbiological circumstances (e.g., 500 mg every 8 to 12 hrs). The recommended dosage in patients with GFR of less than 10 ml/min/1.73 m$^2$ is 250 to 500 mg every 12 hrs, with supplemental doses administered after each dialysis.

**SUGGESTED READINGS**

Hellinger WC, Brewer NS: Imipenem, *Mayo Clin Proc* 66:1074-1081, 1991.
Norrby SR: Carbapenems, *Med Clin North Am* 79:745-759, 1995.

 Does imipenem/cilastatin cross-react with penicillin?

There is a considerable degree of immune cross-reactivity between the penicillins and imipenem, similar to that observed with the cephalosporins. In the initial clinical trials, imipenem was not administered to patients with a history of severe ß-lactam allergy. Imipenem should not be used in patients with immediate hypersensitivity reaction to penicillins (see section under "Allergy").

**SUGGESTED READINGS**

Hellinger WC, Brewer NS: Imipenem, *Mayo Clin Proc* 66:1074-1081, 1991.
Norrby SR: Carbapenems, *Med Clin North Am* 79:745-759, 1995.

# Immunocompromised Host

Q   What empiric antibiotics should be selected for treatment of febrile neutropenic patients?

Febrile patients with neutrophil counts less than 500/µl or those with counts of 500 to 1000/µl in whom a decrease can be anticipated should be assumed to have a potentially life-threatening bacterial infection and promptly treated with broad-spectrum antibiotics by IV route. Before choosing an antibiotic regimen, one should consider the type, frequency of occurrence, and antibiotic susceptibility of bacterial isolates seen in similar patients at his or her hospital.

Several treatment regimens may be considered, including the following:

1. An aminoglycoside (e.g., gentamicin or tobramycin) and antipseudomonal beta-lactam (e.g., ceftazidime, ticarcillin, or piperacillin) should be considered for patients at high risk for *P. aeruginosa* infection (e.g., cancer patients with severe mucositis or those known to be colonized with this organism); major disadvantages include lack of optimal activity against some gram-positive bacteria (e.g., staphylococci) and possible nephrotoxicity and ototoxicity.

2. Combination of two antipseudomonal beta-lactam drugs (e.g., ceftazidime and piperacillin or ticarcillin) should be considered in patients with renal impairment or already on nephrotoxic drugs; disadvantages include selection of resis-

**159**

tant organisms, high cost, possible antagonism of some combinations with certain bacterial isolates, and suboptimal activity against some gram-positive bacteria.

3. Single-drug therapy (e.g., ceftazidime, imipenem/cilastatin) should be considered for patients with neutrophil counts 500 to 1000/μl or brief periods of neutropenia before starting the antibiotic. Close monitoring of patients for lack of response or emergence of drug-resistant organisms is essential, with prompt addition of other broad-spectrum antibiotics as necessary.

4. Vancomycin, aminoglycoside, and antipseudomonal beta-lactam should be considered for patients with suspected methicillin-resistant *S. aureus* infection or with IV catheter–related infection caused by gram-positive organisms.

5. Amphotericin B and broad-spectrum antibiotics should be considered if, after 4 to 7 days of broad-spectrum antibiotic therapy, the fever persists without obvious etiology. This regimen provides additional antifungal coverage (up to 33% of febrile neutropenic patients not responding to a week of antibiotic therapy may have systemic fungal infection, primarily caused by *Candida* or *Aspergillus)*.

Additional considerations include the following:

1. For some patients at low risk of serious complications (e.g., responsive solid tumor with no concurrent comorbidities and with expected neutropenia less than 7 days), less "conventional" (including oral) antibiotic regimens have been successful (see references that follow).

2. Duration of antibiotic therapy is controversial. In the absence of ongoing signs of infection, antibiotics are generally continued until neutrophil count is greater than or equal

to 500/µl or for at least for 5 to 7 days following resolution of fever. If antibiotics are discontinued during neutropenia, close monitoring of the patient for recurrence of fever or the signs of bacterial infection is imperative. Discontinuation of antibiotics in the presence of mucosal lesions, neutrophil count less than 100/µl, and unstable vital signs is *not* recommended.

### SUGGESTED READINGS

Bodey GP: Empirical therapy for fever in neutropenic patients, *Clin Infect Dis* 17(suppl 2):S378-S384, 1993.

Boogaerts MA: Anti-infective strategies in neutropenia, *J Antimicrob Chemother* 36(suppl A):167-178, 1995.

EORTC International Antimicrobial Therapy Cooperative Group: Empiric antifungal therapy in febrile granulocytopenic patients, *Am J Med* 86:668-672, 1989.

Hughes WT et al: Guidelines for the use of antimicrobial agents in neutropenic patients with unexplained fever, *J Infect Dis* 161:381-396, 1990.

Rolston KV, Rubenstein EB, Freifeld A: Early empiric antibiotic treatment for febrile neutropenia patients at low risk, *Infect Dis Clin North Am* 10:223-237, 1996.

How should immunocompromised patients who are exposed to chicken pox be managed?

"Significant" exposure is defined as household contact, face-to-face indoor play, certain exposures within the hospital (same 2- to 4-bed room, adjacent beds in a large ward, face-to-face contact with an infectious staff member or patient for at least 5 minutes, or visit by a person deemed contagious), and newborn infant with onset of varicella in the mother 5 days or less before delivery or within 48 hrs after delivery.

The following persons are candidates for varicella-zoster immune globulin (VZIG) following a significant exposure:

1. Immunocompromised children, adolescents, or adults without history of chicken pox, regardless of VZV antibody test result; some experts do not recommend VZIG administration for children when VZV antibody is detected by a sensitive assay (e.g., FAMA, latex agglutination [LA], or EIA) and the child has not received a blood product that could have provided passive immunity

2. HIV-infected children, adolescents, or adults without history of chicken pox, regardless of VZV antibody test result

3. Susceptible pregnant women (preferably documented by serological testing)

4. Newborn infants whose mothers had onset of chicken pox within 5 days before delivery or within 48 hrs after delivery

5. Hospitalized premature infants (greater than or equal to 28 weeks gestation) whose mothers have no history of chicken pox

6. Hospitalized premature infants (less than 28 weeks gestation or less than or equal to 1000 g), regardless of maternal history

Additional considerations regarding VZIG include the following:

1. Must be given intramuscularly

2. Must be given within 48 hrs of and not more than 96 hrs after exposure (Note: Patients are considered contagious from 1 to 2 days *before* onset of rash; therefore VZIG should often be given within 48 hrs after exposure to a person with varicella rash if significant exposure also occurred during 1 to 2 days before onset of the rash)

3. The duration of protection against chicken pox following VZIG administration is unknown but is usually expected to be no more than 3 weeks

4. The usual adult dose is 5 vials (125 U each)

SUGGESTED READINGS

ACP Task Force on Adult Immunization and Infectious Diseases Society of America: Varicella zoster. In *Guide for adult immunization,* ed 3, Philadelphia, 1994, American College of Physicians.
American Academy of Pediatrics: Varicella-zoster infections. In Peter G, ed: *1994 Red Book: report of the Committee on Infectious Diseases,* ed 24, Elk Grove Village, Ill, 1997, American Academy of Pediatrics.

How should herpes zoster in immunocompromised hosts be treated?

IV acyclovir (10 mg/kg every 8 hrs, assuming normal renal function) for 7 to 10 days is recommended for severely immunocompromised patients with herpes zoster to prevent progression and dissemination of infection. In less profoundly immunocompromised patients, an oral regimen similar to that of immunocompetent patients may be used initially, with close monitoring of the patient's progress.

SUGGESTED READING

Whitley RJ, Gnann JW Jr: Acyclovir: a decade later, *N Engl J Med* 327:782-789, 1992.

What vaccines are contraindicated in immuno-compromised patients?

The Centers for Disease Control and Prevention has proposed categorization of immunocompromised patients into the following three groups for the purpose of receiving live-virus vaccines:

1. Persons who are severely immunocompromised not related to HIV infection (e.g., congenital immunodeficiency, leukemia, lymphoma, generalized malignancy or therapy with alkylating agents, antimetabolites, radiation, or large [usually considered either greater than or equal to 2 mg/kg of body weight or a total of greater than or equal to 20 mg/day of prednisone] amounts of corticosteroids).

Avoid oral polio vaccine (OPV), measles-mumps-rubella (MMR), bacille Calmette-Guérin (BCG), typhoid (live), yellow fever, varicella, and vaccinia.

Note: *Persons with leukemia in remission who have not received chemotherapy for at least 3 months are not considered severely immunosuppressed for the purpose of live-virus vaccination. When cancer chemotherapy or immunosuppressive treatment is being considered, vaccination ideally should precede the initiation of immunosuppressive therapy by at least 2 weeks.*

2. Persons with HIV infection.

Avoid OPV, BCG, typhoid (live), yellow fever, MMR (when CD4 is less than 200), varicella, and vaccinia.

3. Persons with conditions that cause limited immune deficits (e.g., asplenia or renal failure) that may require use of special vaccines or higher doses of vaccines without any contraindication for the use of any particular vaccine.

There is no contraindication to live-virus vaccination.

## VACCINE CONTRAINDICATION CAUSED BY CLOSE CONTACT WITH IMMUNOCOMPROMISED PERSONS

OPV should not be used to immunize patients with immunocompromised household contacts or health care personnel in close contact with immunocompromised patients. If OPV is inadvertently administered to a household or intimate contact of an immunocompromised patient, close contact between the patient and the OPV recipient should be avoided for 1 month after vaccination, the period of maximum excretion of the vaccine virus.

Varicella virus vaccine strain may also be transmitted to household contacts; the manufacturer (Merck) recommends that "vaccine recipients should avoid close association with susceptible high-risk individuals (e.g., newborns, pregnant women, and immunocompromised persons)."

MMR and yellow fever vaccines are not contraindicated in persons with immunocompromised close contacts.

### SUGGESTED READINGS

Centers for Disease Control and Prevention: Recommendations of the Advisory Committee on Immunization Practices (AICP): use of vaccines and immune globulins in persons with altered immunocompetence, *MMWR* 42(RR-4):1-18, 1993.
Centers for Disease Control and Prevention: Update: vaccine side effects, adverse reactions, contraindications, and precautions; recommendations of the Advisory Committee on Immunization Practices (ACIP), *MMWR* 45(RR-12):1-35, 1996.

Hughes P et al: Transmission of varicella-zoster virus from a vaccinee with leukemia, demonstrated by polymerase chain reaction, *J Pediatr* 124:932-935, 1994.

Merck & Co: *Varivax,* March 1995, Manufacturer's package insert.

## STIMULATING QUESTION

Should a patient who previously received isoniazid for 1 year for treatment of a reactive tuberculin skin test receive additional isoniazid therapy after receiving immunosuppressive drugs (e.g., azathioprine)?

Because "preventive" antituberculous therapy is designed to eradicate any remaining potentially infectious *M. tuberculosis* organisms in healed or radiographically invisible lesions, in the absence of reinfection, the protection afforded by such therapy should persist for life. Therefore additional preventive therapy should not be needed regardless of the immunosuppression of the patient.

SUGGESTED READING

American Thoracic Society: Treatment of tuberculosis and tuberculosis infection in adults and children, *Am J Resp Crit Care Med* 149:1359-1374, 1994.

# Influenza

For whom is influenza vaccine indicated?

Influenza vaccine is indicated for the following three major groups of people:

1. High-risk persons (i.e., those at increased risk for influenza-related complications)
   a. Persons 65 years of age or older
   b. Residents of nursing homes and other chronic care facilities housing persons with chronic medical conditions (regardless of age), particularly cardiopulmonary
   c. Adults and children with chronic disorders of the pulmonary or cardiovascular systems, including children with asthma and cystic fibrosis
   d. Adults and children who have required regular medical follow-up or hospitalization during the preceding year because of chronic metabolic diseases (e.g., diabetes mellitus), renal dysfunction, or hemoglobinopathies
   e. Patients with immunosuppression (e.g., HIV or drug-induced)
   f. Children and teenagers (6 months to 18 years of age) who are receiving long-term aspirin therapy and therefore might be at risk for developing Reye's syndrome following influenza
2. Persons who are not necessarily high risk but can transmit influenza to those who are
   a. Physicians, nurses, and other medical and paramedical personnel in hospital and outpatient care settings

**167**

b. Employees of nursing homes and chronic care facilities who have contact with patients or residents
c. Home care providers caring for persons at high risk (e.g., visiting nurses and volunteer workers)
d. Household members (including children) of those in high-risk groups

3. Others
a. Persons who wish to reduce their likelihood of becoming ill with influenza
b. Persons who provide essential community services (e.g., fire fighters and police officers)
c. Students or other persons in institutional settings (e.g., those residing in dormitories)
d. Pregnant women without underlying medical conditions and whose third trimester or early puerperium coincides with the influenza season; there is an increased risk of serious complications from influenza during this period even in the absence of underlying medical conditions

Note: *Influenza vaccination is considered safe during pregnancy.*

e. Pregnant women with underlying medical conditions that increase their risk for complications from influenza
f. Foreign travelers to the tropics at any time of the year and to the southern hemisphere from April through September should receive the most current vaccine preparation

SUGGESTED READINGS

Centers for Disease Control and Prevention: Prevention and control of influenza: recommendations of the Advisory Committee on Immunization Practices (ACIP), *MMWR* 45(RR-5):1-24, 1996.
Kilbourne ED: Inactivated influenza vaccine. In Plotkin SA, Mortimer EA, eds: *Vaccines,* ed 2, Philadelphia, 1994, WB Saunders.

Q When is the best month(s) to receive the influenza vaccine?

Persons at high risk of severe complications from influenza (see previous section) should be offered influenza vaccine beginning each September (when vaccine for the upcoming influenza season becomes available) when they are seen by health care providers for routine care or as a result of hospitalization. Organized vaccination campaigns for persons in high-risk groups should be carried out from October through mid-November.

Vaccination too far in advance of the influenza season (usually peaking between late December and early March in the United States) should be avoided in facilities such as nursing homes because of the potential drop in antibody levels within a few months of vaccination. The vaccine should be offered to children and adults up to and even following when influenza virus activity has been documented in a community. As such, as long as there is a threat of influenza in the community, it is never too late to administer influenza vaccine. In previously unvaccinated children less than 9 years of age, two doses of vaccine are administered 1 month apart, with the second dose administered before December, if possible.

### SUGGESTED READING

Centers for Disease Control and Prevention: Prevention and control of influenza: recommendations of the Advisory Committee on Immunization Practices (ACIP), *MMWR* 45(RR-5):1-34, 1996.

Should a second dose of the influenza vaccine be administered to improve antibody response in adults?

Although influenza vaccine is administered in two doses to children less than 9 years of age without history of influenza vaccination, second dose administration in adults during the same season does not seem to enhance antibody response. Similarly, persons with HIV infection do not seem to have an increased immune response following a second dose of influenza vaccination.

### SUGGESTED READING

Centers for Disease Control and Prevention: Prevention and control of influenza: recommendations of the Advisory Committee on Immunization Practices (ACIP), *MMWR* 45(RR-5):1-24, 1996.

How should amantadine be used for influenza prophylaxis?

Chemoprophylaxis with amantadine (or rimantadine) does not replace the need for vaccination, and it is only effective against influenza A. When used for prophylaxis, amantadine (adults, 100 mg 2×/day if less than 65 years of age, 100 mg 1×/day if 65 years old or older) should be taken daily during the period of ongoing influenza activity in the community. Reported efficacy of amantadine or rimantadine is approximately 70% to 90% in preventing influenza illness (not subclinical infection).

Use of chemoprophylaxis for prevention of influenza is indicated for the following persons at risk of contracting the disease:

- High-risk persons (see previous section) vaccinated after influenza A has begun; administered for 2 weeks in adults and for 6 weeks in children until antibodies develop; does not interfere with the antibody response to the vaccine
- Persons providing care to high-risk persons and vaccinated after influenza A has begun; administered for 2 weeks in adults until antibodies develop
- Persons with immunodeficiency who are expected to have suboptimal antibody response to influenza vaccine (e.g., advanced HIV disease)
- Persons for whom influenza vaccine is contraindicated, including those with severe anaphylactic hypersensitivity reaction to egg protein or other vaccine components
- Persons who wish to avoid influenza A illness; decision should be made on an individual basis

### SUGGESTED READING

Centers for Disease Control and Prevention: Prevention and control of influenza: recommendations of the Advisory Committee on Immunization Practices (ACIP), *MMWR* 45(RR-5):1-24, 1996.

 Does amantadine have a role in the treatment of influenza?

Amantadine (or rimantadine) can reduce the severity and shorten the duration of influenza A illness (not influenza B) among healthy adults when administered within 48 hours of the onset of illness; usual dose is 100 mg 2×/day if less than 65 years of age and 100 mg daily if older than 65 years of age. Duration of treatment is usually 3 to 5 days or within 24 to 48 hrs following resolution of signs and symptoms.

Additional points to remember include the following:

1. Amantadine is cleared primarily by the kidneys; its dosage should be lowered in renal insufficiency (creatinine clearance, 50 ml/min or less)

2. CNS symptoms are not uncommon with the use of amantadine (14%) but appear to be less common with the use of rimantadine (6%)

SUGGESTED READING

Centers for Disease Control and Prevention: Prevention and control of influenza: recommendations of the Advisory Committee on Immunization Practices (ACIP), *MMWR* 45(RR-5):1-24, 1996.

## STIMULATING QUESTION

Does amantadine stop viral shedding when used for the treatment of influenza A infection?

When begun within 48 hours of symptoms in previously healthy adults at a dose of 200 mg/day, amantadine may reduce the duration of viral shedding; it may also decrease the risk of transmission to close contacts. However, persons who have influenza A infection can still shed amantadine- or rimantadine-sensitive viruses early in the course of treatment with these drugs, and they may shed drug-resistant viruses, especially after 5 to 7 days of therapy. They are still capable of transmitting influenza to others with whom they come in contact.

SUGGESTED READINGS

Centers for Disease Control and Prevention: Prevention and control of influenza: recommendations of the Advisory Committee on Immunization Practices (ACIP), *MMWR* 45(RR-5):1-24, 1996.

Tominack RL, Hayden FG: Rimantadine hydrochloride and amantadine hydrochloride use in influenza A virus infections, *Infect Dis North Am* 1:459-478, 1987.

## STIMULATING QUESTION

How do amantadine and rimantadine work against influenza A virus?

The precise mechanism of the antiviral action of amantadine and rimantadine is not clearly defined but appears to be related to the inhibition of an early stage in viral replication, possibly uncoating of the viral genome at the lysosome stage. Attachment and penetration of influenza virus does not appear to be affected by amantadine. Rimantadine also appears to block the intracellular uncoating of influenza viruses.

SUGGESTED READING

Tominack RL, Hayden FG: Rimantadine hydrochloride and amantadine hydrochloride use in influenza A virus infections, *Infect Dis North Am* 1:459-478, 1987.

## STIMULATING QUESTION

Should a person with a history of Guillain-Barré syndrome (GBS) receive influenza vaccine?

Unlike the 1976 swine influenza vaccine, subsequent vaccine preparations of other influenza viral strains have not clearly been associated with GBS. Although the incidence of GBS in the general population is extremely low, persons with a history of this disease have a substantially greater likelihood of subsequent development of GBS than those without such a history. Whether influenza vaccination is causally associated with this risk for recurrence is not known.

The Centers for Disease Control and Prevention states that "although it would seem prudent to avoid a subsequent influenza vaccination in a person known to have developed GBS within 6 weeks of a previous influenza vaccination, for most persons with a history of GBS who are at high risk for severe complications from influenza, the established benefits of influenza vaccination justify yearly immunization."

SUGGESTED READING

Centers for Disease Control and Prevention: Prevention and control of influenza: recommendations of the Advisory Committee on Immunization Practices (ACIP), *MMWR* 45(RR-5):1-24, 1996.

# Lactobacillus

Q What is the significance of growth of *Lactobacillus* sp. from "clean-catch" urine specimens?

Lactobacilli are an important part of the normal bacterial flora of man and are ordinarily found in large numbers in the intestine and female genitourinary tract (i.e., the vagina, periurethral area, and urethra of postpubertal women). Lactobacilli are the predominant vaginal organisms in 80% to 90% of normal women. They are considered among the least pathogenic of the bacteria associated with humans and are often referred to as "friendly anaerobes"; serious infections are extremely rare.

Lactobacilli may be isolated from the midstream urine of up to 35% of asymptomatic women, with 12% to 20% of women having concentrations of 10,000/ml of organisms in pure culture. In symptomatic women with dysuria, up to 66% of first-stream specimens may contain high counts of lactobacilli; however, when suprapubic urinary samples are obtained in these women, no lactobacilli are usually found.

Given these findings and the inherent low virulence of these organisms, *lactobacilli isolated from "clean-catch" urine specimens should generally not be considered urinary pathogens and do not require antibiotic treatment.* In fact, overgrowth of lactobacilli in the vagina or distal urethra is often a complication of prior therapy with antimicrobial agents that have little or no in vitro activity against these organisms (e.g., trimethoprim-sulfamethoxazole). Whether lactobacilli can cause dysuria or "urethral syndrome" in women as a result of overgrowth in the urethra without affecting the bladder or upper urinary tract remains controversial.

### SUGGESTED READINGS

Bokkenheuser V: The friendly anaerobes, *Clin Infect Dis* 16(suppl 4):S427-S434, 1993.

Gillespie WA et al: Microbiology of the urethral (frequency and dysuria) syndrome. A controlled study with 5-year review, *Br J Urol* 64:270-274, 1989.

Hamilton-Miller JMT, Brumfitt W, Smith GW: Are fastidious organisms an important cause of dysuria and frequency? The case against. In Asscher AW, Brumfitt W, eds: *Microbial diseases in nephrology,* New York, 1986, John Wiley & Sons.

Maskell R: Are fastidious organisms an important cause of dysuria and frequency? The case for. In Asscher AW, Brumfitt W, eds: *Microbial diseases in nephrology,* New York, 1986, John Wiley & Sons.

Maskell R: A new look at the diagnosis of infection of the urinary tract and its adjacent structures, *J Infect* 19:207-217, 1989.

 What antibiotics are effective in the treatment of infections caused by lactobacilli?

Rarely, lactobacilli may cause serious infections (e.g., bacteremia, wound infection, endocarditis, septic arthritis, abdominal/pelvic abscess, peritonitis, endometritis, or amnionitis) that require antimicrobial therapy. Lactobacilli are uniformly susceptible in vitro to penicillin G or ampicillin, carbenicillin, and chloramphenicol. Clindamycin has activity against 94% of isolates, erythromycin against 88%, tetracycline against 60%, metronidazole against 50%, and cephalosporins against 89% to 95%. Some strains are also resistant to vancomycin. Trimethoprim-sulfamethoxazole has no appreciable activity against lactobacilli (see previous question).

*A significant discrepancy between the minimum inhibitory concentration and the minimum bactericidal concentration is observed in some isolates; in these cases, use of a potentially synergistic combination of drugs, such as penicillin G and an aminoglycoside, should be considered.*

## SUGGESTED READINGS

Bayer AS et al: Lactobacillemia—report of nine cases; important clinical and therapeutic considerations, *Am J Med* 64:808-813, 1978.

Brook I, Frazier EH: Significant recovery of nonsporulating anaerobic rods from clinical specimens, *Clin Infect Dis* 16:476-480, 1993.

Hamilton-Miller JMT, Brumfitt W, Smith GW: Are fastidious organisms an important cause of dysuria and frequency? The case against. In Asscher AW, Brumfitt W, eds: *Microbial diseases in nephrology*, New York, 1986, John Wiley & Sons.

# Legionnaires' Pneumonia

Q How can legionnaires' pneumonia be diagnosed?

Although none of the signs or symptoms of legionnaires' pneumonia are specific to this disease, the following clues should raise the possibility of legionnaires' pneumonia:

1. Gram stain of respiratory secretions showing many neutrophils but few, if any, organisms. *Legionella* sp. is either not seen on gram stain or appears as small, pleomorphic, faintly staining, gram-negative rods.

2. Hyponatremia (serum sodium less than 130 mEq/ml). This electrolyte abnormality occurs significantly more frequently (17% to 47%) in legionnaires' disease than in pneumonias of other etiologies.

3. Lack of response to beta-lactam antibiotics (penicillin or cephalosporin) and aminoglycosides.

4. Pneumonia diagnosed in a hospital or environment in which the potable water supply is known to be contaminated with *Legionella* sp.

However, because none of the previously mentioned features are specific for legionnaires' pneumonia, specific laboratory tests are necessary for definitive diagnosis; these include culture, direct fluorescent antibody stain, antibody detection, DNA probe, and urinary antigen.

**178**

Urinary antigen test has a sensitivity of 80% and a specificity of 99%. Although it detects only *Legionella pneumophila* serogroup 1, the latter accounts for 80% to 90% of clinically apparent legionnaires' pneumonia cases. Its advantages also include the ability to obtain rapid results, occasional difficulty obtaining sputum sample in critically ill patients, its relative low cost, and persistence of a positive test for days or months during or after the administration of antibiotics.

Culture of *Legionella* sp. from clinical specimens such as respiratory secretions is the definitive method for diagnosis of legionnaires' pneumonia. Specimens obtained by bronchoscopy are useful but do not necessarily provide a higher yield than an appropriately obtained sputum sample (sensitivity 80%). Transtracheal aspirate has a sensitivity of 90%. If sputum is not available, bronchoalveolar lavage may be used; bronchial wash specimens give lower yield. Because standard bacteriological media do not adequately support the growth of *Legionella* sp., a buffered charcoal yeast extract agar is usually used as base media. The laboratory personnel should be notified of the need to specifically culture for *Legionella*. The organisms grow slowly and require usually 3 to 5 days before colonies on the agar can be spotted macroscopically. Blood cultures, when appropriately obtained and processed for *Legionella* sp., have a reported sensitivity of 20% to 38%. Previous antimicrobial therapy may affect the yield of cultures.

Direct fluorescent antibody is performed directly on specimens and has a reported sensitivity of 25% to 80%, depending on the quantity of organisms in the specimen, and a specificity of 96% to 99%.

DNA probe/hybridization tests for *Legionella* ribosomal RNA are genus specific and have a sensitivity comparable to that of direct fluorescent antibody test.

Serological testing for detection of *Legionella*-specific antibodies has become less useful with the advent of more rapid tests and cultures. Four to twelve weeks may be required to detect an antibody response, rendering this test not helpful in making an immediate diagnosis of legionnaires' disease. A fourfold rise in antibody titer or the presence of IgM and IgG antibodies is supportive of the diagnosis. Sensitivity ranges from 40% to 60%, with a specificity of 96% to 99%. Highest specificity is for *L. pneumophila* serogroup 1; testing for antibodies to other serogroups or *Legionella* sp. is discouraged.

Note: *Regardless of the method of diagnosis, every attempt must be made to culture Legionella from clinical specimens because of the high specificity of cultures and the need for serotyping of the isolate for epidemiological purposes.*

### SUGGESTED READINGS

Edelstein PH: Legionnaire's disease, *Clin Infect Dis* 16:741-749, 1993.
Nguyen MH, Stout JE, Yu VL: Legionellosis, *Infect Dis Clin North Am* 5:561-584, 1991.
Yu VL: *Legionella pneumophila* (legionnaire's disease). In Mandell GL, Bennett JE, Dolin R, eds: *Principles and practices of infectious diseases*, ed 4, New York, 1995, Churchill Livingstone.

 What is the best treatment for legionnaires' pneumonia?

High-dose erythromycin (1 g every 6 hrs IV) has traditionally been considered the initial antibiotic of choice based on clinical experience rather than controlled trials. Major drawbacks of high-dose erythromycin therapy include ototoxicity (observed in up to 20% of patients, but reversible) and the need for large-volume fluid administration. It is recommended that high-dose erythromycin be given to those patients with immunosuppression or severe pneumonia; others may respond equally as well to a dose of 500 mg every 6 hrs.

Because of its excellent in vitro activity and intracellular penetration, rifampin 600 mg 2×/day is often added in cases of more severe legionnaires' disease (e.g., respiratory failure or multilobar pneumonia) and in patients with severe immunosuppression. Lung damage is less severe in animals that are administered rifampin with or without erythromycin, but survival is not significantly different in this setting.

Other drugs reported to be effective include trimethoprim-sulfamethoxazole (5 mg of trimethoprim component per kg IV every 8 hrs), ciprofloxacin (400 mg IV every 8 to 12 hrs), clarithromycin (500 mg 2×/day), and azithromycin (500 mg daily). There is no apparent synergy between fluoroquinolones and rifampin experimentally. Anecdotal reports of efficacy of tetracyclines (e.g., doxycycline and minocycline) can also be found in the literature. Despite a report of successful treatment with imipenem, this drug, as well as other beta-lactam antibiotics (e.g., penicillin and cephalosporins), should *not* be used for treatment of legionnaires' disease because of their low macrophage concentrations and generally poor clinical response. Similarly, aminoglycoside should not be used for treatment of legionnaires' pneumonia.

Optimal duration of therapy is not known, although 10 to 21 days is usually recommended; however, immunosuppressed patients may require longer course of therapy. Clinical response usually occurs within 3 to 5 days of adequate treatment. Once desirable clinical response has been achieved, a switch from parenteral to oral antibiotic therapy is appropriate. Chest radiograph is not useful for determining clinical response and by itself should not be used to determine the mode or duration of therapy.

## SUGGESTED READINGS

Edelstein PH: Imipenem in legionnaire's disease, *Lancet* 2:757, 1984.

Edelstein PH: Legionnaire's disease, *Clin Infect Dis* 16:741-749, 1993.

Nguyen MH, Stout JE, Yu VL: Legionellosis, *Infect Dis Clin North Am* 5:561-584, 1991.

Unertl KE et al: Ciprofloxacin in the treatment of legionellosis in critically ill patients including those cases unresponsive to erythromycin, *Am J Med* 87(suppl 5A):128S-131S, 1989.

Yu VL: *Legionella pneumophila* (legionnaire's disease). In Mandell GL, Bennett JE, Dolin R, eds: *Principles and practices of infectious diseases,* ed 4, New York, 1995, Churchill Livingstone.

# Lower Respiratory Tract Infections

 **Q** What is the best way to treat *P. aeruginosa* respiratory tract infections?

For treatment of *P. aeruginosa* pneumonia, a combination of an antipseudomonal penicillin (e.g., piperacillin, ticarcillin, and mezlocillin), ceftazidime, aztreonam, or imipenem and an aminoglycoside (e.g., tobramycin, gentamicin, and amikacin) is generally recommended. Although ciprofloxacin has good in vitro activity against *P. aeruginosa*, its use as monotherapy for pneumonia caused by this organism is not recommended (67% failure to achieve bacteriological eradication and 33% rate of development of resistance). Whenever possible, selection of antibiotics should be based on in vitro susceptibility data. Duration of treatment is usually 3 weeks or longer.

In patients with clinically stable cystic fibrosis and endobronchial *P. aeruginosa* infection, tobramycin 600 mg in 30 ml of half-strength physiological saline 3×/day by ultrasonic nebulizer for 28 days has been found to be efficacious and safe.

## SUGGESTED READINGS

Chastre J, Fagon JY, Trouillet JL: Diagnosis and treatment of nosocomial pneumonia in patients in intensive care units, *Clin Infect Dis* 21(suppl 3):S226-S237, 1995.

Fink MP et al: Treatment of severe pneumonia in hospitalized patients: results of multicenter, randomized, double-blind trial comparing intravenous ciprofloxacin with imipenem-cilastatin, *Antimicrob Agents Chemother* 38:547-557, 1994.

Korvick JA, Yu VL: Antimicrobial agent therapy for *Pseudomonas aeruginosa, Antimicrob Agents Chemother* 35:2167-2172, 1991.
Ramsey BW et al: Efficacy of aerosolized tobramycin in patients with cystic fibrosis, *N Engl J Med* 328:1740-1746, 1993.

What is the treatment of choice for *H. influenzae* respiratory tract infection?

Whenever possible, antibiotic selection should be based on in vitro susceptibility data. In the United States, resistance of *H. influenzae* to ampicillin (rate of 20% to 40%), erythromycin, cephalexin, cefadroxil, and cephradine is common. Resistance to cefaclor, cefprozil, loracarbef, and tetracycline has been reported in 1% to 5% clinical isolates. Resistance to cefuroxime, cefixime, amoxicillin/clavulanate, trimethoprim-sulfamethoxazole, azithromycin, clarithromycin, and quinolones has been found in less than 1% of clinical isolates.

For serious respiratory tract infections (e.g., pneumonia and epiglottitis), cefotaxime, ceftriaxone, and cefuroxime are appropriate. For upper respiratory tract infections and bronchitis, an oral antibiotic with predictable in vitro activity (see previous discussion) may be chosen.

### SUGGESTED READINGS

Anonymous: The choice of antibacterial drugs, *Med Lett Drugs Ther* 38:25-34, 1996.
Doern GV: Trends in antimicrobial susceptibility of bacterial pathogens of the respiratory tract, *Am J Med* 99(suppl 6B):3S-7S, 1995.

Q  What is the recommended treatment for *S. aureus* pneumonia?

*S. aureus* pneumonia in previously healthy adults is rare, except following influenza infections. Antibiotic selection should be based on in vitro susceptibility data. Community-acquired (excluding nursing homes) *S. aureus* isolates are usually susceptible to semisynthetic penicillins (e.g., nafcillin or oxacillin) and first-generation cephalosporins (e.g., cefazolin). In the absence of resistance to oxacillin, therapy should be initiated with maximal doses of one of these agents. Bacteriostatic drugs such as erythromycin or tetracycline should be avoided. Similarly, clindamycin should not be considered a first-line agent. Patients allergic to penicillins and cephalosporins should be treated with IV vancomycin. For severe infections, the addition of gentamicin or rifampin should be considered.

In the case of methicillin-resistant *S. aureus* (MRSA) pneumonia, vancomycin either alone or in combination with gentamicin or rifampin is the agent of choice.

Treatment should be continued for a minimum of 2 weeks. Even in the presence of adequate treatment, defervescence may be slow. Persistence of moderately elevated temperatures for 1 to 2 weeks is not uncommon.

## SUGGESTED READINGS

Blinkhorn RJ Jr: Community-acquired pneumonia. In Baum GL, Wolinsky E, eds: *Textbook of pulmonary disease,* ed 5, Boston, 1994, Little, Brown.

Waldvogel FA: *Staphylococcus aureus* (including toxic shock syndrome). In Mandell GL, Bennett JE, Dolin R, eds: *Principles and practices of infectious diseases,* ed 4, New York, 1995, Churchill Livingstone.

What is the recommended treatment for *N. meningitidis* lower respiratory tract infections, and should household members receive chemoprophylaxis?

*N. meningitidis* is a recognized cause of pneumonia. Treatment of choice is penicillin G; alternatively, ceftriaxone, cefotaxime, or chloramphenicol may be used. Empiric use of sulfonamides should be avoided because of high prevalence of resistance to these drugs among *N. meningitidis* isolates. Duration of antibiotic therapy may vary, but 10 to 14 days appears reasonable.

Chemoprophylaxis of household members is recommended following diagnosis of any invasive meningococcal infection, including pneumonia. The drug of choice in most instances is rifampin 600 mg orally every 12 hrs for 2 days for adults (remember *two* [300-mg] pills, 2×/day, for 2 days), and 10 mg/kg (maximum dose 600 mg) every 12 hrs for 2 days for children (older than 1 month of age).

For pregnant women, ceftriaxone 250 mg IM is indicated. Ciprofloxacin 500 mg as a single dose has also been effective in eradicating meningococcal carriage in adults; it is not recommended for use in persons younger than 18 years of age.

### SUGGESTED READINGS

American Academy of Pediatrics: Meningococcal infections. In Peter G, ed: *1997 Red Book: report of the Committee on Infectious Diseases,* ed 24, Elk Grove Village, Ill, 1997, American Academy of Pediatrics.

Apicella MA: *Neisseria meningitidis.* In Mandell GL, Bennett JE, Dolin R, eds: *Principles and practices of infectious diseases,* ed 4, New York, 1995, Churchill Livingstone.

What is the best treatment for *Acinetobacter* spp. lower respiratory tract infections?

Most pulmonary infections caused by *Acinetobacter* occur nosocomially, with prior antibiotic therapy and residence in the intensive care unit (ICU) found to be significant risk factors. Increasingly, *Acinetobacter* has become resistant to numerous antibiotics in many centers. Antibiotic selection should be based on in vitro susceptibility data.

Most *A. baumanni* are resistant to ampicillin and cefotaxime, with some centers reporting up to 91% of nosocomial *Acinetobacter* resistant to gentamicin. For severe infections, a combination of an effective beta-lactam (e.g., ticarcillin, piperacillin, ceftazidime, or imipenem/cilastatin) and an aminoglycoside (e.g., amikacin or tobramycin) is often recommended. Fluoroquinolones (e.g., ciprofloxacin) may also be effective, but rapid emergence of resistance when used as monotherapy may pose a problem. Trimethoprim-sulfamethoxazole may also be effective.

### SUGGESTED READING

Allen DM, Hartman BJ: *Acinetobacter* species. In Mandell GL, Bennett JE, Dolin R, eds: *Principles and practices of infectious diseases,* ed 4, New York, 1995, Churchill Livingstone.

 What is the best treatment for *Enterobacter* respiratory tract infections?

As with many other etiological agents of nosocomial pneumonia, *Enterobacter* infections often occur in the setting of prior antibiotic therapy in hospitalized patients. *Enterobacter* isolates are commonly resistant to first-generation cephalosporins (e.g., cefazolin or cephalexin) and develop antibiotic resistance to second- and third-generation cephalosporins (e.g., cefuroxime or ceftazidime) caused by an inducible beta-lactamase enzyme.

Antibiotic selection should take into account the in vitro susceptibility data. Treatment with antipseudomonal penicillins (e.g., ticarcillin, piperacillin), imipenem, or ciprofloxacin with or without an aminoglycoside is often recommended.

## SUGGESTED READINGS

Eisenstein BI: Enterobacteriaceae. In Mandell GL, Bennett JE, Dolin R, eds: *Principles and practices of infectious diseases,* ed 4, New York, 1995, Churchill Livingstone.

Fussle R et al: Development of resistance by *Enterobacter cloacae* during therapy of pulmonary infections in intensive care patients, *Clin Invest* 72:1015-1019, 1994.

# Lyme Disease

Q How is Lyme disease transmitted?

*B. burgdorferi,* the spirochete agent of Lyme disease, is transmitted by the bite of ticks of Ixodes family. The nymphal stage is primarily responsible for transmission of the disease. In experimental studies, tick attachment for 24 hours or more is necessary before transmission of the spirochete occurs. Following injection of *B. burgdorferi* by the tick, it may spread locally in the skin (erythema migrans) or in the blood or lymph to other sites. Virulent strains of *B. burgdorferi* may resist elimination by phagocytic cells initially, and the immune response may be suppressed.

### SUGGESTED READING

Steere AC: Borrelia burgdorferi (Lyme disease, Lyme borreliosis). In Mandell GL, Bennett JE, Dolin R, eds: *Principles and practices of infectious diseases*, ed 4, New York, 1995, Churchill Livingstone.

Q How should Lyme disease serologies be interpreted?

Lack of standardization and interlaboratory differences in testing have plagued *B. burgdorferi* serology. Screening serological tests include indirect ELISA, IFA, and antibody-capture EIA. In patients with indeterminate or positive responses, Western blotting or immunoblotting may be performed for confirma-

**189**

tion. False-positive serological tests may be associated with polyclonal B-cell activation, positive rheumatoid factor and antinuclear antibody, active infectious mononucleosis, and syphilis. False-negative antibody tests can be seen in localized disease (e.g., erythema migrans) and in cases associated with early treatment. Even specific IgM response to *B. burgdorferi* does not peak until 3 to 6 weeks after onset of disease.

Note: *Because of the possibility of asymptomatic or past infection, a positive* B. burgdorferi *antibody by itself is not diagnostic of active symptomatic Lyme disease. Serologies should always be interpreted in the context of clinical history and patient signs and symptoms.*

**SUGGESTED READINGS**

Steere AC: Borrelia burgdorferi (Lyme disease, Lyme borreliosis). In Mandell GL, Bennett JE, Dolin R, eds: *Principles and practices of infectious diseases,* ed 4, New York, 1995, Churchill Livingstone.
Weil HFC, Franck WA, Hardin JA: Lyme disease (tick-borne borreliosis). In Reese RE, Betts RF, eds: *A practical approach to infectious diseases,* Boston, 1991, Little, Brown.

 How should Lyme disease be treated?

For early local (erythema migrans) and disseminated Lyme disease, doxycycline 100 mg 2×/day, amoxicillin 500 mg 4×/day, cefuroxime axetil 500 mg 2×/day, or azithromycin 500 mg daily seems to be effective. Duration of treatment is 10 to 21 days. For late-stage Lyme disease with CNS or joint involvement (arthritis), parenteral ceftriaxone (2 g daily), cefotaxime (2 g 3×/day), or penicillin G (5 million U 4×/day) for 3 to 4 weeks is often used.

## SUGGESTED READING

Steere AC: Borrelia burgdorferi (Lyme disease, Lyme borreliosis). In Mandell GL, Bennett JE, Dolin R, eds: *Principles and practices of infectious diseases,* ed 4, New York, 1995, Churchill Livingstone.

Q   Should all tick bites be treated with prophylactic antibiotics for Lyme disease?

Even in areas in which Lyme disease is endemic, the risk of infection with *B. burgdorferi* after a tick bite is usually so low that routine prophylaxis following tick bites is unnecessary, probably because of the relatively long (24 hours or more) duration of tick attachment necessary for transmission of infection. In cases associated with engorged ticks, unpredictable patient follow-up, pregnancy, or highly anxious patients, prophylactic antibiotics may be considered in endemic areas. Either amoxicillin or doxycycline (in nonpregnant persons or children older than 8 years) for 10 days may be effective in preventing Lyme disease.

## SUGGESTED READINGS

Shapiro ED et al: A controlled trial of antimicrobial prophylaxis for Lyme disease after deer-tick bites, *N Engl J Med* 327:1769, 1992.
Steere AC: Borrelia burgdorferi (Lyme disease, Lyme borreliosis). In Mandell GL, Bennett JE, Dolin R, eds: *Principles and practices of infectious diseases,* ed 4, New York, 1995, Churchill Livingstone.
Weil HFC, Franck WA, Hardin JA: Lyme disease (tick-borne borreliosis). In Reese RE, Betts RF, eds: *A practical approach to infectious diseases,* Boston, 1991, Little, Brown.

## STIMULATING QUESTION

What is the risk of transmission of Lyme disease to a surgeon operating on a patient with erythema migrans?

*B. burgdorferi* isolation from blood occurs rarely even in patients thought to have disseminated disease. Not surprisingly, no cases of transfusion-related or occupationally acquired Lyme disease have ever been reported.

SUGGESTED READING

Nadelman RB et al: Isolation of *Borrelia burgdorferi* from the blood of seven patients with Lyme disease, *Am J Med* 88:21-26, 1990.

# Malaria Prophylaxis

 When is malaria prophylaxis indicated for overseas travel, and what drugs can be used?

Travelers to areas of the world with malaria are advised to use an appropriate drug regimen and personal protection measures to reduce (but not necessarily eliminate) their risk of acquiring malaria.

Malaria transmission occurs in large parts of Central and South America, Hispaniola, sub–Saharan Africa, the Indian subcontinent, Southeast Asia, the Middle East, and Oceania. The risk of acquiring malaria varies significantly from area to area and is dependent on the intensity of transmission within the various areas, the itinerary, and the time and type of travel. Even in the same area within a country, the risk of malaria increases when considerable time is spent in rural areas and during evenings and nighttime hours. For example, tourists who travel to urban areas and stay in air-conditioned hotels may be at lower risk of acquiring malaria than backpackers or adventure travelers who spend considerable amounts of time outdoors.

The appropriate chemoprophylactic regimen is dependent on whether the travelers will be at risk of acquiring drug-resistant *Plasmodium falciparum*. The following is a list of the countries with reported malaria according to the chemoprophylactic regimen recommended by the Centers for Disease Control and Prevention (December 1996).

**193**

## COUNTRIES WITH AREAS FOR WHICH MEFLOQUINE PROPHYLAXIS IS INDICATED

Afghanistan

Angola

Bangladesh (all areas, except no risk in Dhaka)

Benin

Bhutan (rural areas, in districts bordering India)

Bolivia (rural areas, except no risk in highland areas [Oruro Department, Province of Ingavi, Los Andes, Omasuyos, Pacajes-La Paz Department, Southern and central Potosi Department])

Botswana (northern part of country [north of 21° latitude south])

Brazil (Acre and Rondonia states; territories of Amapa and Roraima; part of rural areas of the following states: Amazona, Maranhao, Mato Grosso, Pará, Tocantins, outskirts of Manaus and Porto Velho) (Note: Travelers who will visit only the coastal states from the horn to the Uruguay border and Iguassu Falls are not at risk and need no prophylaxis.)

Burkina Faso

Burma (see Myanmar)

Burundi

Cambodia (all, except no risk in Phnom Penh; western provinces, doxycycline)

Cameroon

Central African Republic

Chad

China (rural areas of southern China, Hainan Island, provinces bordering Myanmar, Lao People's Democratic Republic, and Vietnam; north of 33° latitude north, transmission occurs July to November; from 33° latitude north to 25° latitude north, transmission occurs May to December; south of 25° latitude north, transmission occurs year round; no risk in northern provinces bordering Mongolia and in the western provinces of Heilungkiang, Kirin, Ningsia Hui Tibet, and Tsinghai; travelers visiting cities and popular rural sites on usual tourist routes are generally not at risk, and chemoprophylaxis is therefore not recommended; travelers on special scientific, educational, or recreational visits should check whether their itineraries include evening or nighttime exposure in areas of risk or in areas of chloroquine resistance)

Colombia (rural areas only of Alto Vaupes [Vaupes Comisaria], Amazonas, Ariari [Meta Department], Bajo Cauca-Nechi [Cauca and Antioquia Department], Caqueta [Caqueta Intendencia], Catatumbo [Norte de Santander Department], Guainia [Comisarias], Magdalena Medio, Pacifico Central and Sur Putumayo [Putumayo Intendencia], Sarare [Aruca Intendencia], Urabá [Antioquia Department]; no risk in Bogota and vicinity)

Comoros

Congo

Cote d'Ivoire (formerly Ivory Coast)

Djibouti

Ecuador (all provinces along eastern border and Pacific coast; travelers who will visit only Quito and vicinity, the central highland tourist areas, or the Galapagos Islands are not at risk and need no prophylaxis)

Equatorial Guinea

Eriteria (all, except no risk at altitudes higher than 2000 m)

Ethiopia (all, except no risk in Addis Ababa and at altitudes higher than 2000 m)

French Guinea

Gabon

Gambia

Ghana

Guinea

Guinea-Bissau

Guyana (rural, in all interior regions including Rupununi and northwest regions and areas along Pomeroon River)

India (all, including the cities of Delhi and Bombay, except no risk in parts of states of Himechel [Pradesh], Jammu, Kashmir, and Sikkim)

Indonesia (rural only, except high risk in all areas of Irian Jaya [western half of island of New Guinea]; no risk in cities of Java and Sumatra and no risk for the main resort areas of Java and Bali; chemoprophylaxis is recommended only for travelers who will have outdoor exposure during evening and nighttime hours in rural areas)

Iran-Islamic Republic (rural only in the provinces of Sistan-Baluchestan; the tropical part of Kerman; Hormozgan, parts of Bushehr, Fars, and Ilam; Kohgiluyeh-Boyar; Lorestan; Chahar Mahal-Bakhtiari; and the north of Khuzestan)

Kenya (all, including game parks, except no risk in Nairobi and at altitudes higher than 2500 m)

Lao People's Democratic Republic (all, except no risk in city of Vientiane)

Liberia

Madagascar (highest risk in coastal areas)

Malawi

Malaysia (peninsular Malaysia and Sarawak [northwest Borneo]: malaria limited to remote areas; urban and coastal areas: malaria free; Sabah [northeast Borneo]: malaria throughout; chemoprophylaxis is recommended only for travelers who will have outdoor exposure during evening and nighttime hours in rural areas)

Mali

Mauritania (all areas, except no risk in the northern region: Adrar, Dakhlet-Nouadhibou, Inchiri, and Tiris-Zemour)

Mayotte (French territorial collectively)

Mozambique

Myanmar (rural areas only; travelers who visit the cities of Yangon [formerly Rangoon] and Mandelay are not at risk and need no prophylaxis; chemoprophylaxis is recommended only for travelers who will have outdoor exposure during evening and nighttime hours in rural areas)

Namibia (all Ovamboland and Caprivi Strip)

Nepal (rural in Terai District and Hill Districts below 1200 m; no risk in Katmandu)

Niger

Nigeria

Oman

Pakistan (all areas below 2000 m, including the cities)

Panama (areas east of the Canal Zone, including the San Blas Islands)

Papua New Guinea

Peru (rural areas of provinces bordering Brazil and Ecuador; chemoprophylaxis recommended for travelers who will have rural exposure during evening and nighttime hours; travelers who will visit only Lima and vicinity, coastal areas south of Lima, or the highland tourist areas [Cuzco, Machu Picchu, and Lake Titicaca] are not at risk and need no prophylaxis)

Philippines (islands of Basilian, Luzon, Mindanao, Mindoro, Palawan, Sulu-Archipelago; chemoprophylaxis is recommended only for travelers who will have outdoor exposure during evening and nighttime hours in rural areas)

Rwanda

Sao Tome and Principe

Senegal

Sierra Leone

Solomon Islands

Somalia

South Africa (rural areas, including game parks, in the northern, eastern, and western low-altitude areas of Transvaal and in the Natal coastal areas north of 28° latitude south)

Sri Lanka (risk in all rural areas; no risk in the districts of Colombo, Kalutara, and Nuwara Eliya)

Sudan

Suriname (rural areas only, except no risk in Paramaribo District and coastal areas north of 5° latitude north)

Swaziland (all lowlands)

Tanzania-United Republic of

Togo

Uganda

Vanuatu (formerly New Hebrides; all areas except no risk on Fortuna Island)

Venezuela (rural areas, in all border states and territories and the states of Barinas, Merida, and Portugesa)

Vietnam (rural only, except no risk in the Red River Delta and the coastal plain north of Nha Trang)

Yemen (all areas, except no risk in Aden and airport perimeter)

Zaire

Zambia

Zimbabwe (all, except no risk in cities of Harare and Bulawayo)

## COUNTRIES WITH AREAS FOR WHICH CHLOROQUINE PROPHYLAXIS IS INDICATED

Note: *Mefloquine prophylaxis may be indicated for certain areas of the following countries listed.*

Argentina (rural areas near Bolivian border [i.e., Salta and Jujuy provinces] and along border with Parquay [i.e., Misiones and Corrientes provinces])

Azerbaijan (very small areas of southern border)

Belize (rural areas including forest preserves, offshore islands, and resort areas; no risk in central coast District of Belize)

China *(see also section under mefloquine prophylaxis)* (rural areas not covered under section on mefloquine prophylaxis; no risk in northern provinces bordering Mongolia and in the western provinces of Heilungkiang, Kirin, Ningsia Hui Tibet, and Tsinghai; north of 33° latitude north, transmission occurs July to November; from 33° latitude north to 25° latitude north, transmission occurs May to December; south of 25° latitude north, transmission occurs year round; no risk in northern provinces bordering Mongolia and in the western provinces of Heilungkiang, Kirin, Ningsia Hui Tibet, and Tsinghai; travelers visiting cities and popular rural sites on usual tourist routes are generally not at risk, and chemoprophylaxis is therefore not recommended; travelers on special scientific, educational, or recreational visits should check whether their itineraries include evening or nighttime exposure in areas of risk)

Costa Rica (rural areas only [including tourist areas], except no risk in central highlands [i.e., Cartago and San Jose Provinces])

Dominican Republic (rural areas, except no risk in tourist resorts; highest risk in provinces bordering Haiti)

Egypt (El Faiyum area; travelers visiting main tourist areas, including cruises, are not at risk and need no prophylaxis)

El Salvador (rural areas only)

Guatemala (rural areas only, except no risk in central highlands)

Haiti

Honduras (rural only)

Iraq (all northern provinces of Duhok, Erbil, Ninawa, Sulaimaniya, Támim, and Basrah)

Mauritius (rural areas only, except no risk on Rodrigues Island)

Mexico (rural areas of the following states: Campeche, Chiapas, Guerrero, Michoacan, Nayarit, Oaxaca, Quintana Roo, Sinaloa, and Tabasco)

Nicaragua (rural areas only; however, risk exists in outskirts of Bluefields, Bonanza, Chinandega, Leon, Puerto Cabeza, Rosita, and Siuna)

Panama *(see also section under mefloquine prophylaxis)* (rural areas west of the Canal Zone; no risk in the Canal Zone, Panama city, and vicinity)

Paraguay (rural areas only, bordering Brazil)

Peru *(see also section under mefloquine prophylaxis)* (rural areas not covered under section on mefloquine resistance; chemoprophylaxis recommended for travelers who will have rural exposure during evening and nighttime hours; travelers who will visit only Lima and vicinity, coastal areas south of Lima, or the highland tourist areas [Cuzco, Machu Picchu, and Lake Titicaca] are not at risk and need no prophylaxis)

Philippines *(see also section under mefloquine resistance)* (rural areas not covered under section on mefloquine prophylaxis; chemoprophylaxis is recommended only for travelers who will have outdoor exposure during evening and nighttime hours in rural areas)

Saudi Arabia (all of western provinces, except no risk in the high-altitude areas of Asir province [Yemen border] and the urban areas of Jeddah, Mecca, Medina, and Taif)

Syrian Arab Republic (rural areas only, except no risk in southern and western districts of Deir-es-zor and Sweida)

Tajikistan (southern border only)

Turkey (southeast Anatolia and Cukorova/Amikova areas only)

United Arab Emirates (northern emirates except no risk in Emirate of Abu Dhabi or in cities of Ajman, Dubai, Sharjah, and Umm al Qaiwan)

## COUNTRIES WITH AREAS FOR WHICH DOXYCYCLINE PROPHYLAXIS IS INDICATED

Cambodia *see also section under mefloquine prophylaxis)* (western provinces; no malaria risk in Phnom Penh)

Thailand (limited risk with malaria largely confined to forested rural areas, principally along the borders with Cambodia and Myanmar, not visited by most travelers; most travel to rural areas in Thailand is during daytime hours when the risk of exposure is minimal; no risk of malaria in cities and major tourist resorts [e.g., Bangkok, Chiangmai, Pettaya, and Phuket])

## ADULT DOSAGE REGIMEN FOR COMMONLY PRESCRIBED ANTIMALARIAL DRUGS USED FOR PROPHYLAXIS

Mefloquine (Lariam) 228-mg base (250-mg salt) PO, 1×/week, to be started 1 to 2 weeks before travel to malarious area and continued for 4 weeks after leaving such an area

Chloroquine phosphate (Aralen) 300 mg base (500 mg salt) PO, 1×/week, to be started 1 to 2 weeks before travel to malarious area and continued for 4 weeks after leaving such an area

Doxycycline 100 mg PO 1×/day, to be started 1 to 2 days before travel to malarious area and continued for 4 weeks after leaving such an area

## SUGGESTED READING

Centers for Disease Control and Prevention: *Health information for international travel 1996-97,* December 1996, US Department of Health and Human Services, Public Health Service.

 What are some concerns and side effects associated with the use of antimalarial drugs used for prophylaxis?

*For complete list of adverse effects, physicians should review the product package insert.*

Mefloquine: Rarely associated with severe reactions such as psychosis and convulsions; minor side effects include gastrointestinal disturbance, insomnia, and dizziness. The frequency of reported symptoms declines with increasing duration of prophylaxis, and the drug may be better tolerated when taken in the evening.

*Contraindications/precautions:* Known hypersensitivity to mefloquine, history of epilepsy or severe psychiatric disorders, pregnancy or possibility of pregnancy within 2 months (may be considered after the first trimester if travel to an area with intense transmission of chloroquine-resistant *P. falciparum* is anticipated), children who weigh less than 15 kg, chronic hepatic dysfunction, history of cardiac conduction abnormalities (may be used in persons concurrently on beta blockers, if they have no underlying arrhythmia); package insert cautions against use of the drug by drivers, pilots, and machine operators because of concerns about spatial disorientation and motor coordination; caution is also advised with the use of mefloquine in scuba divers because of the risk of neurological symptoms developing at depth and the similarities of symptoms of decompression illness (dizziness, headache, nausea, and fatigue) with those of mefloquine; should be used with caution in patients with psychiatric disturbances because it has been associated with emotional disturbances; concomitant administration with quinine or chloroquine may increase the risk of convulsions.

Chloroquine: Rarely causes serious adverse reaction when used at prophylactic doses for malaria; minor side effects include gastrointestinal disturbance, headache, dizziness, blurred vision, and pruritus, but generally these effects do not require discontinuation of the drug; may exacerbate psoriasis; may interfere with the antibody response to human diploid cell rabies vaccine when the vaccine is administered intradermally; not recommended for persons with preexisting retinal macular degeneration; periodic eye examinations recommended for long-term users; considered safe during pregnancy.

Doxycycline: May cause photosensitivity, usually manifested as an exaggerated sunburn reaction; risk lower by avoiding prolonged, direct exposure to the sun and by using sunscreens that absorb long-wave ultraviolet (UVA) radiation; associated with an increased frequency of monilial vaginitis; gastrointestinal side effects (nausea or vomiting) may be minimized by taking the drug with a meal; should not be taken before going to bed to reduce risk of esophagitis.

*Contraindications:* Pregnant or nursing mothers and children less than 8 years of age.

## SUGGESTED READINGS

Centers for Disease Control and Prevention: *Health information for international travel 1996-97,* December 1996, US Department of Health and Human Services, Public Health Service.

Jong EC, White NJ: Malaria prevention. In Jong EC, McCullen R, eds: *The travel & tropical medicine manual,* Philadelphia, 1995, WB Saunders.

*Physician's desk reference,* ed 51, Montvale, NJ, 1997, Medical Economics.

# Meningitis

 How should "aseptic/viral meningitis" be diagnosed?

Enteroviruses (e.g., echovirus and coxsackievirus A and B) are the most common cause of aseptic meningitis, accounting for more than 80% of cases for which an etiology can be identified. Other causes include mumps, lymphocytic chorimeningitis (LCM) virus, herpesvirus, HIV, cytomegalovirus, EBV, influenza A and B virus, parainfluenza, arthropod-borne viruses, and adenovirus.

Headache, fever, malaise, pharyngitis, nausea, vomiting, and meningismus are common. The peripheral white blood count is usually not helpful. The cerebrospinal fluid (CSF) leukocyte count is usually less than 500/ml but occasionally is higher. Although lymphocytic pleocytosis is common, early in the disease a polymorphonuclear predominance may be seen (in up to two thirds of the enteroviral cases), which will often shift to mononuclear predominance on follow-up lumbar puncture over the following 6 to 48 hours. The CSF protein is usually normal or mildly elevated (<100 mg/dl), and CSF glucose is typically normal.

Enterovirus infections are found more commonly during the warmer months but may be seen year round. Enteroviruses have been reported to be isolated from CSF in about 40% to 80% of cases (the author's experience suggests much lower rate of recovery in adults, however). Because of lack of widely available rapid diagnostic tests for enteroviral infections and lack of specific therapy, the diagnosis of enteroviral meningitis is often presumptive. The isolation of enterovirus from throat or stool is suggestive rather than diagnostic of enteroviral infection because viral shedding may occur for weeks after infection and in healthy controls.

Mumps meningitis is most common during late winter and spring in temperate climates. CSF parameters are often similar to those found in enteroviral meningitis, except that low CSF glucose has been found in up to 25% of mumps meningitis. Diagnosis is often made by acute and convalescent serology. Mumps virus may be grown from CSF.

LCM virus is transmitted to humans by contact with rodents (mice or hamsters) or their excreta and is often diagnosed in late fall and early winter. The peripheral leukocyte and platelet count may be decreased, but CSF leukocyte counts may occasionally be in the thousands. CSF glucose is low in up to 25% of cases. Diagnosis is often made by acute and convalescent serology.

Of the herpesviruses, herpes simplex type 2 has been most frequently associated with aseptic meningitis in adults, usually occurring in the setting of primary genital infection. Meningitis is less common with recurrent genital herpes. Diagnostic methods include CSF cultures, serology, and, most recently, PCR.

HIV may be a cause of aseptic meningitis at the time of initial infection and seroconversion. Diagnosis is suggested by serological testing or detection of HIV antigen or RNA (e.g., by PCR) in the serum.

Arthropod-borne viruses (e.g., California encephalitis, St. Louis encephalitis, and Eastern and Western equine encephalitis viruses) usually cause encephalitis but, in their milder forms, may be associated with aseptic meningitis. They are more common during warmer months, and their presentations may be indistinguishable from those of enteroviral meningitis. Epidemiological clues such as the time of the year and abundance of mosquitoes in the area may be helpful. Diagnosis is usually made by acute and convalescent serology.

### SUGGESTED READINGS

Connolly KJ, Hammer SM: The acute aseptic meningitis syndrome, *Infect Dis Clin North Am* 4:599-622, 1990.

Tedder DG et al: Herpes simplex virus infection as a cause of benign recurrent lymphocytic meningitis, *Ann Intern Med* 121:334-338, 1994.

 How should viral meningitis be managed?

Treatment of viral meningitis is usually supportive. Headache and nausea should be adequately controlled with appropriate analgesics and antiemetics. IV fluids should be administered to patients with poor oral intake and vomiting. In patients with herpes simplex–associated meningitis, treatment with acyclovir is reasonable. Patients with acute HIV infection syndrome may benefit from antiretroviral therapy as it relates to their clinical course and CD4 cell count.

### SUGGESTED READINGS

Bergstrom T, Alestig K: Treatment of primary and recurrent herpes simplex virus type 2 induced meningitis with acyclovir, *Scand J Infect Dis* 22:239-240, 1990.

Connolly KJ, Hammer SM: The acute aseptic meningitis syndrome, *Infect Dis Clin North Am* 4:599-622, 1990.

Kinloch-De Loes S et al: A controlled trial of zidovudine in primary human immunodeficiency virus infection, *N Engl J Med* 333:408-413, 1995.

Q What infection control guidelines are recommended for hospitalized patients with enteroviral meningitis? What about their household contacts?

These viruses are transmitted by direct contact with nose and throat discharges and feces and by aerosol droplets. Therefore measures to minimize such contact should be implemented. In the hospital, standard/enteric precautions should suffice and strict hand washing after patient contact should be enforced. Similarly, household members should avoid contact with the patient's respiratory secretions and feces and should be encouraged to wash their hands frequently. There is no role for testing of asymptomatic contacts, and no chemoprophylaxis is available.

### SUGGESTED READING

Benenson AS: Coxsackievirus diseases, *Control of communicable diseases manual*, ed 6, Washington, DC, 1995, American Public Health Association.

Q What chemoprophylactic regimen should be used for prevention of bacterial meningitis?

There are two types of bacterial meningitis for which chemoprophylaxis of contacts is indicated: meningococcal and *H. influenzae* type B (Hib) meningitis.

## MENINGOCOCCAL MENINGITIS

Household, child care center, and nursery school contacts of patients with invasive meningococcal infection should receive chemoprophylaxis as soon as possible, preferably within 24 hours of the diagnosis of the primary case. Prophylaxis is also recommended for persons who have had contact with the patient's oral secretions through kissing or sharing of food or beverages. Health care workers usually do not require prophylaxis unless they have had intimate exposure (e.g., mouth-to-mouth resuscitation, intubation, or suctioning) before appropriate therapy was begun. There is no role for respiratory tract cultures in determining who should receive chemoprophylaxis. Rifampin (10 mg/kg, maximum per dose 600 mg, 2×/day for 2 days) is the drug of choice (remember the rule of "2s"—two pills, 2×/day, for 2 days). Alternatively ciprofloxacin 500 mg as a single dose or ceftriaxone (125 mg for children younger than 12 years; 250 mg for children older than 12 years old and for adults) may be considered; the latter is a particularly attractive option for pregnant females.

## HIB MENINGITIS

The following persons should be considered for chemoprophylaxis after exposure to a case of Hib meningitis:

1. All household contacts (regardless of age) where there is at least one person younger than 4 years of age (unvaccinated, or vaccinated but immunocompromised). Contacts who spent at least 4 hrs with the index patient for at least 5 of the 7 days preceding the day of hospital admission of the index patient are managed similar to household contacts. Prophylaxis is not recommended for pregnant contacts because of uncertain effect of rifampin on the fetus.

2. Child care and nursery school contacts under circumstances when unvaccinated or incompletely vaccinated children younger than 2 years also attend the center for 25 hrs/week or more. When two or more cases of invasive Hib

occur among attendees within 60 days and unvaccinated or incompletely vaccinated children attend the center, chemoprophylaxis should also be recommended to all attendees and supervisory personnel.

Rifampin is the chemoprophylactic agent of choice and is administered at 20 mg/kg (600 mg for adults) once daily PO for 4 days. Although rifampin should be administered as soon as possible following diagnosis of infection in the index case, it may still be of some benefit when initiated 7 or more days after such diagnosis.

Note: *The index case should also receive rifampin prophylaxis just before hospital discharge, except for those treated with cefotaxime or ceftriaxone.*

### SUGGESTED READINGS

American Academy of Pediatrics: *Haemophilus influenzae* infections. In Peter G, ed: *1997 Red Book: report of the Committee on Infectious Diseases,* ed 24, Elk Grove Village, Ill, 1997, American Academy of Pediatrics.
American Academy of Pediatrics: Meningococcal infections. In Peter G, ed: *1997 Red Book: report of the Committee on Infectious Diseases,* ed 24, Elk Grove Village, Ill, 1997, American Academy of Pediatrics.

## STIMULATING QUESTION

A 32-weeks' gestation pregnant female was exposed to a patient subsequently diagnosed to have meningococcal meningitis. What prophylaxis should be used?

If exposure is considered significant (see previous section), prophylaxis with ceftriaxone (250 mg IM) is reasonable as long as there are no contraindications to its use. Ciprofloxacin is contraindicated during pregnancy, and the effect of rifampin on the fetus has not been well established.

## SUGGESTED READING

American Academy of Pediatrics: Meningococcal infections. In Peter G, ed: *1997 Red Book: report of the Committee on Infectious Diseases,* ed 24, Elk Grove Village, Ill, 1997, American Academy of Pediatrics.

## STIMULATING QUESTION

Should a health care worker who performed mouth-to-mouth resuscitation on an untreated patient with pneumococcal meningitis receive any kind of chemoprophylaxis?

Currently, there are no recommendations for chemoprophylaxis of pneumococcal meningitis.

## SUGGESTED READING

Benenson AS: *Control of communicable diseases manual,* ed 16, Washington, DC, 1995, American Public Health Association.

# Mycoplasma pneumoniae

 What is the treatment of choice for *Mycoplasma* pneumonia?

Erythromycin at 500 mg PO 4×/day and tetracyclines (e.g., doxycycline 100 mg 2×/day or tetracycline 500 mg 4×/day) are equally effective in the treatment of *M. pneumoniae* in adults. Both reduce the duration of respiratory tract symptoms, but because of up to 10% relapse rate, treatment should be continued for 3 weeks.

Clarithromycin, azithromycin, and quinolones (e.g., ciprofloxacin and ofloxacin) should also be effective but are much more costly. It should be noted that antibiotics do not eliminate the carrier state, possibly because of the persistence of organisms intracellularly. Because of the lack of a cell wall, cell wall–active antibacterial agents such as penicillins and cephalosporins are ineffective.

## SUGGESTED READINGS

Baum SG: *Mycoplasma pneumoniae* and atypical pneumonia. In Mandell GL, Bennett JE, Dolin R, eds: *Principles and practices of infectious diseases,* ed 4, New York, 1995, Churchill Livingstone.

Martin RE, Bates JH: Atypical pneumonia, *Infect Dis North Am* 5:585-601, 1991.

How should *Mycoplasma* serology be interpreted?

The most diagnostically useful serological testing for acute *Mycoplasma* infection is *M. pneumoniae*–specific IgM by indirect immunofluorescence or ELISA because its presence usually indicates recent infection. False-positive results may occur in the presence of acute pancreatitis, possibly related to the cross-reaction between pancreatic tissue and mycoplasmal lipid antigen.

Alternatively, a fourfold or greater rise in *Mycoplasma* antibody titers (found in serum samples obtained late in the course of the illness) by complement fixation supports the diagnosis. Cold-agglutinin titers greater than or equal to 1:64 also suggest *Mycoplasma* infection; however, it is only 50% sensitive and may be positive in other infections such as influenza, infectious mononucleosis, psittacosis, rubella, adenovirus, cytomegalovirus infection, and lymphoma.

**SUGGESTED READINGS**

Baum SG: *Mycoplasma pneumoniae* and atypical pneumonia. In Mandell GL, Bennett JE, Dolin R, eds: *Principles and practices of infectious diseases,* ed 4, New York, 1995, Churchill Livingstone.

Martin RE, Bates JH: Atypical pneumonia, *Infect Dis Clin North Am* 5:585-601, 1991.

# Needlestick/Blood and Body Fluid Exposure

 How should needlestick exposures at the workplace be managed?

The major steps in managing puncture injuries related to contaminated sharps in the health care setting are as follows:

1. Wound care
   a. Routine wound/splash cleansing
   b. Provide tetanus immunization (Td) if 5 years or greater since last vaccination
2. Source person serological evaluation
   a. Test for HbsAg, HCV antibody
   b. Test for HIV antibody with patient/guardian's informed consent
   c. If the source is unknown, assess for likelihood of presence of blood-borne viral infection; if there is a significant likelihood of source having blood-borne viral infection, manage exposed person as if he or she were exposed to these agents
3. Hepatitis B evaluation/prophylaxis following significant/ percutaneous exposure
   a. Exposed person serological evaluation
      ▪ Baseline: HbsAg, anti-HbsAg, ALT/AST (SGPT/SGOT); anti-HbsAg optional if exposed known to have adequate titers within the last 24 months
      ▪ Follow-up: HbsAg, anti-HbsAg, anti-HBc, ALT/AST in 3 and 6 months
   b. Prophylaxis (Table 2)

TABLE 2    *Recommendations for postexposure hepatitis B prophylaxis*

| Exposed person status | Treatment when source is found to be | | Unknown or untested |
|---|---|---|---|
| | HbsAg + | HbsAg − | |
| Unvaccinated | HBIG* ×1 and HBV vaccine series | HBV vaccine series | HBV vaccine series |
| Previously vaccinated | | | |
| Known responder | Test exposed person for anti-HbsAg†: 1. If adequate, no treatment 2. If inadequate, HBV vaccine booster | No treatment | No treatment |
| Known nonresponder | HBIG ×2 or HBIG ×1 and HBV vaccine ×1 | No treatment | If known high-risk,‡ may treat as if source were HbsAg positive |
| Response unknown | Test exposed person for anti-HBsAg: 1. If adequate, no treatment 2. If inadequate, HBIG ×1 and HBV vaccine booster | No treatment | Test exposed person for anti-HBsAg: 1. If adequate, no treatment 2. If inadequate, hepatitis B vaccine booster dose |

*Hepatitis B immune globulin IM 0.06 mg/kg (maximum 5 ml) should be given as soon as possible after exposure and within 24 hrs, if possible. The value of HBIG administration more than 7 days postexposure is unclear. It should be given at a separate site if given simultaneously with HBV vaccine.

†Adequate defined as >10 milli-international units.

‡High-risk individuals include those from areas with HBV endemicity and their descendants (e.g., China, Southeast Asia, most of Africa, most Pacific Islands, parts of Middle East, Amazon Basin, and Alaskan natives), users of illicit parenteral drugs, sexually active homosexual men, male prisoners, clients in instituions for the developmentally disabled, household contacts and sexual partners of HBV carriers, hemodialysis patients, and heterosexuals with multiple partners.

4. Hepatitis C evaluation/prophylaxis following significant/ percutaneous exposure
   a. Exposed person serological evaluation
      - Baseline: anti-HCV, ALT/AST
      - Follow-up: anti-HCV, ALT/AST at 3 and 6 months
   b. Prophylaxis: none recommended
5. HIV evaluation/prophylaxis following significant/percutaneous exposure (see section under "HIV")

SUGGESTED READINGS

Centers for Disease Control and Prevention: The hepatitis B virus: a comprehensive strategy for eliminating transmission in the United States through universal childhood vaccination, *MMWR* 40:1-25, 1991.

Koziol DE, Henderson DK: Nosocomial viral hepatitis in health care workers. In Mayhall CG, ed: *Hospital epidemiology and infection control,* Baltimore, 1996, Williams & Wilkins.

## STIMULATING QUESTION

*An immunocompetent laboratory worker stuck her finger with a needle contaminated with active M. tuberculosis cultures. What should she do?*

Intact skin is relatively resistant to exogenous mycobacterial infection. However, cutaneous tuberculosis as a result of puncture injury to the skin has been reported in laboratory workers and other health care workers. Pathogenesis of cutaneous tuberculosis from an exogenous inoculation is similar to that of primary pulmonary disease, with initial multiplication of mycobacteria causing an ulcer (tuberculous chancre) or nodule composed of nonspecific inflammatory cells within 3 weeks followed by lymphatic extension and regional lymphadenopathy 3 to 6 weeks after inoculation. The purified protein derivative (PPD) skin test becomes reactive. The prognosis has been favorable in the majority of cases regardless of therapy.

There are no known published protocols for management of health care workers with puncture injuries involving *M. tuberculosis*. Specifically, there are no recommendations regarding routine chemoprophylaxis in this setting before documentation of tuberculosis infection either based on cutaneous manifestation or PPD skin test conversion. Nevertheless, the following course of action seems reasonable.

Standard local care of the injured skin should be administered, and the exposed health care worker should undergo PPD skin testing soon after the accident, with repeat testing 2 to 3 months following inoculation (if not previously known or found to have positive skin test). The exposed person should be closely followed for signs of local inflammation, nodule, or ulcer at the site of puncture, with excisional biopsy and appropriate cultures performed to document possible mycobacterial infection. Optimal treatment of primary cutaneous tuberculosis is not known, although a 6-month regimen consisting of isoniazid, rifampin, and pyrazinamide for drug-sensitive organisms seems reasonable.

### SUGGESTED READINGS

Beyt BE: Cutaneous tuberculosis. In Schlossberg D, ed: *Clinical topics in infectious diseases: tuberculosis*, New York, 1988, Springer-Verlag.

Kramer F et al: Primary cutaneous tuberculosis after a needlestick injury from a patient with AIDS and undiagnosed tuberculosis, *Ann Intern Med* 119:594-595, 1993.

## STIMULATING QUESTION

A veterinarian accidentally punctures himself with a needle used for *Brucella* vaccine in cattle. What should be done?

The commonly used bovine *Brucella* vaccines are based on live-attenuated preparations and are capable of producing febrile disease in humans. Although there are no clinical studies, prophylactic use of doxycycline 200 mg/day PO for 6 weeks, concomitantly with rifampin 300 mg 3×/day for the first 30 days is often recommended by the Missouri Department of Health.

## SUGGESTED READINGS

Nicoletti P: *Vaccination against* Brucella: *bacterial vaccines,* New York, 1990, Alan R Liss.

Satalowich FT: Personal communication, 1996, Bureau of Veterinary Public Health, Missouri Department of Health.

Yound EJ: Brucellosis. In Hoeprich PD, Jordan MC, Ronald AR, eds: *Infectious diseases,* ed 5, Philadelphia, 1994, JB Lippincott.

# Nontuberculous Mycobacteria

 How should the growth of nontuberculous mycobacteria from a sputum culture be interpreted, and when is treatment recommended?

In contrast to tuberculosis, in which the isolation of a single colony of *M. tuberculosis* from sputum is always clinically significant, nontuberculous mycobacteria may colonize the respiratory tract without necessarily causing disease. In addition, because of their ubiquitous nature (found in soil, water, and dust), they may frequently contaminate clinical specimens. Thus at times the differentiation between contamination, colonization, and disease may be problematic. Treatment is appropriate if disease is likely. Colonization alone without the presence of disease is not a sufficient reason for treatment of nontuberculous mycobacteria.

The American Thoracic Society has adopted the following guidelines for the diagnosis of pulmonary *disease* caused by nontuberculous mycobacteria (1990):

1. For patients with cavitary lung disease
   a. Presence of two or more sputum specimens (or sputum and a bronchial washing) that are acid-fast bacilli smear-positive or result in moderate-to-heavy growth of nontuberculous mycobacteria on culture
   b. Other reasonable causes for pulmonary disease have been excluded (e.g., tuberculosis and fungal disease)

218

2. For patients with noncavitary lung disease
   a. Presence of two or more sputum specimens (or sputum and a bronchial washing) that are smear-positive for acid-fast bacilli or produce moderate-to-heavy growth on culture
   b. If the isolate is *Mycobacterium kansasii* or *M. avium* complex, failure of the sputum cultures to clear with bronchial toilet or within 2 weeks of institution of specific mycobacterial drug therapy (this criterion is probably also valid for other species of nontuberculous mycobacteria)
   c. Other reasonable causes for the pulmonary disease process have been excluded
3. For patients with cavitary or noncavitary lung disease whose sputum evaluation is nondiagnostic or another disease cannot be excluded
   a. A transbronchial or open lung biopsy yields the organism and shows mycobacterial histopathological features (i.e., granulomatous inflammation, with or without acid-fast bacilli); other criteria are not needed
   b. A transbronchial or open lung biopsy that fails to yield the organism but shows mycobacterial histopathological features in the absence of a history of other granulomatous or mycobacterial disease *and* (1) presence of two or more positive cultures of sputum or bronchial washings and (2) exclusion of other reasonable causes for granulomatous lung disease
4. In patients with AIDS, respiratory secretions demonstrating growth of nontuberculous mycobacteria in association with evidence of dissemination (e.g., positive blood or bone marrow cultures)

Additional considerations in deciding whether to treat a nontuberculous mycobacterium isolate from respiratory secretions include the following:

1. The species of *Mycobacterium* isolated is important. Certain species are rarely, if ever, associated with human disease (e.g., *M. gordonae),* whereas other species are rarely environmental contaminants (e.g., *M. kansasii).*
2. The quantity of growth of cultures of respiratory secretions is important. "Heavy growth" is usually associated with disease, whereas scant growth is likely to represent colonization or contamination.
3. The majority of patients with nontuberculous mycobacterial pulmonary disease have chronic underlying lung disease (e.g., pneumoconioses associated with silicosis and coal mining, healed chronic infections such as tuberculosis and mycosis, chronic bronchitis and emphysema, and bronchiectasis) as a predisposing factor, possibly related to impaired local protective mechanisms (e.g., bronchopulmonary clearance).
4. Immunological state of the host should always be considered. Relatively "avirulent" nontuberculous mycobacteria may be more likely to cause disease in immunosuppressed patients.
5. History may provide clues regarding the type of mycobacterial infection:
   a. Achalasia of the esophagus associated with chronic regurgitation or from those who ingest mineral oil: consider *M. fortuitum* complex
   b. Coal miner: *M. kansasii*
   c. Severe hemoptysis: *M. fortuitum* complex
   d. Institutional outbreak: *M. xenopi*
   e. Chronic pulmonary disease with recurrent pneumonia, especially in older women: *M. avium* complex

## SUGGESTED READINGS

Horowitz EA, Sanders WE Jr: Other mycobacterium species. In Mandell GL, Bennett JE, Dolin R, eds: *Principles and practices of infectious diseases,* ed 4, New York, 1995, Churchill Livingstone.
O'Brien RJ: The epidemiology of nontuberculous mycobacterial disease, *Clin Chest Med* 10:407-418, 1989.

Raszka WV Jr et al: Isolation of nontuberculous, non-avium mycobacteria from patients infected with human immunodeficiency virus, *Clin Infect Dis* 20:73-76, 1995.

Wallace RJ Jr et al: Diagnosis and treatment of disease caused by nontuberculous mycobacteria (official statement ATS), *Am Rev Resp Dis* 142:940-953, 1990.

Wolinsky E: Mycobacterial diseases other than tuberculosis, *Clin Infect Dis* 15:1-10, 1992.

## STIMULATING QUESTION

What type of mycobacterial infection can one get from exposure of abraded skin to swimming pool water, and how should it be treated?

Swimming pool granuloma is caused by *M. marinum* and can present in two clinical forms: (1) localized nodular form with solitary or multiple lesions that may undergo suppuration or ulceration and scaling and (2) lymphatic form similar to sporotrichosis. It is thought that the lesion occurs as a result of inoculation of the mycobacterium into the skin by trauma. Involvement of underlying tissues and systemic signs and symptoms are rare, possibly related to the inability of the organism to grow optimally at body temperature. The incubation period is usually 2 to 8 weeks. Most cases of *M. marinum* infection heal spontaneously, but lesions may persist for months. Standard chlorination of swimming pools should prevent growth of this organism.

Recommended treatment when indicated includes two-drug combination (e.g., ethambutol and rifampin, and clarithromycin and ethambutol or rifabutin). Monotherapy with tetracyclines, minocycline, doxycycline, trimethoprim-sulfamethoxazole, or clarithromycin has also been advocated. Deeper infections often involve a combination of medical therapy and surgical excision of the infected tissue. Duration of antibiotic treatment is usually a minimum of 3 months.

## SUGGESTED READINGS

Dalovisio JR, Pankey GA: Dermatologic manifestations of nontuberculous mycobacterial diseases, *Infect Dis Clin North Am* 8:677-688, 1994.

Garty B: Swimming pool granuloma associated with erythema nodosum, *Cutis* 47:314-316, 1991.

Guay DR: Nontuberculous mycobacterial infections, *Ann Pharmacother* 30:819-830, 1996.

# Osteomyelitis

 How can osteomyelitis in the foot of a diabetic patient with a draining wound be diagnosed?

The foot should be examined carefully, and sinus tracts should be probed to identify infections extending to the bone. Palpation of bone in the depths of infected foot ulcers is strongly correlated with the presence of underlying osteomyelitis (sensitivity 66%, specificity 85%, positive predictive value 89%, and negative predictive value 56%). If bone is palpated on probing, specialized roentgenographic and radionuclide testing is usually not necessary for diagnosis of contiguous focus osteomyelitis. In contrast, if the extent of the infection cannot be determined at the bedside, radiographic imaging may be helpful.

Note: *It should be stressed that no imaging technique has perfect sensitivity and specificity. Therefore interpretation of these tests should take into account the patient's clinical history and setting.*

The imaging process should usually start with the plain radiograph, which has a reported sensitivity of 28% to 93% and a specificity of 50% to 92% for detecting osteomyelitis; the latter is often related to noninfectious osteopathy, which may also be associated with cortical defects close to joints and osteolysis. Because plain radiography may be negative early in the infection, it should be repeated in 2 to 4 weeks when osteomyelitis is suspected.

**223**

Three-phase technetium bone scan is generally very sensitive (70% to 100%) but has suboptimal specificity (less than 50% in several studies) for diagnosis of osteomyelitis (neuropathic changes in the foot may also show positive results). Thus, although a negative bone scan is helpful in excluding osteomyelitis, a positive result does not necessarily support this diagnosis.

Indium-111 leukocyte scan has good sensitivity (75% to 100%) but may be associated with false-positive results (specificity 73% to 89%); it cannot differentiate progressive neuropathic joint from an infected joint.

Magnetic resonance imaging (MRI) is generally considered to have high sensitivity and specificity for diagnosis of osteomyelitis in diabetic foot infections; sensitivity is usually greater than 90%, and specificity ranges from 75% to 90%.

In summary, in evaluating a diabetic foot ulcer for the possibility of underlying osteomyelitis, it should initially be probed to determine bone involvement. If the wound does not appear to involve the bone, a plain radiograph should be obtained. If the radiograph is highly suggestive of osteomyelitis, surgical exploration with culture of the bone should be considered. On the other hand, if the radiograph is not supportive of a diagnosis of suspected osteomyelitis, an MRI scan should be considered to exclude bone marrow changes as well as deep tissue abscesses. Other imaging modalities should be performed possibly as an adjunct to MRI scan if there are lingering doubts about the possibility of underlying osteomyelitis, taking into account their potential limitations.

### SUGGESTED READINGS

Brower AC: What is the preferred method for diagnosing osteomyelitis in the foot of a patient with diabetes? *AJR* 163:471-472, 1994.

Eckman MH et al: Foot infections in diabetic patients: decision and cost-effectiveness analyses, *JAMA* 273:712-720, 1995.

Grayson ML et al: Probing to bone in infected pedal ulcers: a clinical sign of underlying osteomyelitis in diabetic patients, *JAMA* 273:721-723, 1995.

Lipsky BA, Pecoraro RE, Wheat LJ: The diabetic foot: soft tissue and bone infection, *Infect Dis Clin North Am* 4:409-432, 1990.

Longmaid HE III, Kruskal JB: Imaging infections in diabetic patients, *Infect Dis Clin North Am* 9:163-182, 1995.

How should osteomyelitis associated with diabetic foot ulcers be managed?

Inadequate diagnosis or treatment of osteomyelitis in a diabetic patient with foot ulcer increases the risk for amputation. Osteomyelitis should always be considered in the presence of diabetic foot ulcer, with one third to two thirds of patients with moderate or severe infections having underlying osteomyelitis in this setting.

Surgical treatment should always be considered for all diabetic foot osteomyelitis for diagnostic (including culture of bone) and therapeutic purposes (e.g., débridement of necrotic bone and drainage of potential deep-seated abscess). Gangrenous infections, necrotizing fasciitis, or other life-threatening deep-seated infections require immediate amputation.

Antimicrobial therapy should be based on the isolated organisms from bone cultures (should be performed aerobically and anaerobically). Superficial cultures of the wound usually produce results that overrepresent the true pathogenic flora causing bone infection (total concordance 27%). "Reliable" cultures likely to represent bone isolates are likely to yield a single organism, whereas "unreliable" cultures are more likely to yield four or more organisms. Selection of antimicrobial agents based on surface cultures will cover appropriate pathogens in 93% of cases (62% appropriate, 31% excessive spectrum) and is inadequate in 8% of cases. *S. aureus,* coagulase-negative staphylococci, streptococci, anaerobes, and aerobic gram-negative bacilli (e.g., *Proteus* sp., *P. aeruginosa)* are common isolates. Empiric initial therapy with a broad-spectrum cephalosporin and an antibiotic active against anaerobes (e.g., metronidazole or clindamycin) or with an extended-spectrum penicillin (e.g., piperacillin-tazobactam, ticarcillin/clavulanate, or ampicillin-sulbactam) is a reasonable choice. Antibiotic combination therapy with aminoglycosides is usually reserved for patients with resistant gram-negative bacilli or *P. aeruginosa* infection. Parenteral antibiotics are usually used in the initial phase of treatment of osteomyelitis (usually for at least 4 weeks) followed by oral antibiotics. Oral quinolones (e.g., ciprofloxacin or ofloxacin) hold promise in shortening the duration of or replacing parenteral antibiotics in the treatment of osteomyelitis caused by aerobic gram-negative bacilli. The duration of antimicrobial therapy should be based on the specific patient's clinical response but usually is several weeks (minimum 2 to 3 months). Expert consultation should be obtained.

## SUGGESTED READINGS

Bamberger DM, Daus GP, Gerding DN: Osteomyelitis in the feet of diabetic patients: long term results, prognostic factors, and the role of antimicrobial and surgical therapy, *Am J Med* 83:653-660, 1987.

Grayson ML: Diabetic foot infections. Antimicrobial therapy, *Infect Dis Clin North Am* 9:143-161, 1995.

Lipsky BA, Pecoraro RE, Wheat LJ: The diabetic foot; soft tissue and bone infection, *Infect Dis Clin North Am* 4:409-432, 1990.

Vibhagool A, Calhoun J, Mader JP: Therapy of bone and joint infections, *Hosp Formul* 28:63-85, 1993.

Wheat LJ et al: Diabetic foot infections: bacteriologic analysis, *Arch Intern Med* 146:1935-1940, 1986.

Q     How should osteomyelitis associated with pressure sores be diagnosed?

Most pressure sores are *not* associated with underlying osteomyelitis. Neither clinical parameters (e.g., duration of ulcer, bone exposure, purulent drainage, and fever) nor laboratory data (e.g., peripheral white blood cell count and erythrocyte sedimentation rate) are helpful in identifying patients who have underlying osteomyelitis. For example, in one study only 14% of decubitus ulcers associated with visible bone were found to have underlying osteomyelitis.

Plain roentgenograms have poor sensitivity and specificity and therefore should not be relied on to diagnose or exclude osteomyelitis in this setting. Specifically, radiographic changes often associated with osteomyelitis, such as lucencies, periosteal changes, and sclerosis, are also frequently found in biopsy-negative bone specimen obtained from underneath decubitus ulcers.

Three-phase bone scan is highly sensitive (nearly 100%) but has very poor specificity (as low as 7%) in patients with decubitus ulcers. Thus whereas a negative bone scan essentially excludes the presence of underlying osteomyelitis, a positive scan is poorly predictive of this diagnosis (less than 20%).

The role of other radiographic tests such as gallium scan, indium-labeled leukocyte scintigraphy, CT, and MRI in diagnosing osteomyelitis associated with decubitus ulcers has not been well defined.

Currently, bone biopsy (either by needle or open surgical technique) is considered the only standard criterion for diagnosis of osteomyelitis underlying pressure ulcers. Culture of the ulcer is of no value in predicting causative organisms of underlying osteomyelitis.

## SUGGESTED READINGS

Darouiche RO et al: Osteomyelitis associated with pressure sores, *Arch Intern Med* 154:753-758, 1994.

Sugarman B: Pressure sores and underlying bone infection, *Arch Intern Med* 147:553-555, 1987.

Thornhill-Joynes M et al: Osteomyelitis associated with pressure ulcers, *Arch Phys Med Rehabil* 67:314-318, 1986.

 How should osteomyelitis associated with decubitus ulcers be managed?

Infected and devitalized bone should be surgically excised. When indicated, transposition of a well-perfused musculocutaneous flap is often recommended to promote a rapid decrease in the local bacterial concentration and enhancement of host defenses against infection.

A 4- to 6-week course of antibiotic therapy is commonly recommended, although treatment for longer than 3 weeks does not appear to affect the outcome of the patient. Theoretically, when all infected bone is removed, long-term antibiotics should not be necessary. Selection of antibiotics should be based on bone cultures whenever possible. Potential pathogens include enteric gram-negative bacteria such as *E. coli*, anaerobes, *Pseudomonas* sp., and *Staphylococcus* sp.

## SUGGESTED READINGS

Baack BR: Pressure ulcers. In Fry DE, ed: *Surgical infections,* Boston, 1995, Little, Brown.

Darouiche RO et al: Osteomyelitis associated with pressure sores, *Arch Intern Med* 154:753-758, 1994.

Thornhill-Joynes M et al: Osteomyelitis associated with pressure ulcers, *Arch Phys Med Rehabil* 67:314-318, 1986.

# Parotitis

How should acute parotitis be treated?

Acute parotitis may have viral or bacterial causes. Viral parotitis may be caused by a variety of agents, including paramyxovirus (mumps), influenza A virus, parainfluenza viruses, EBV, and enteroviruses (e.g., coxsackieviruses). Treatment is generally symptomatic and consists of relief of pain and fever and prevention of dehydration. Patients should be closely monitored for secondary bacterial infection.

Acute bacterial parotitis often affects elderly, malnourished, dehydrated, and postoperative patients. In addition to parotid swelling and tenderness, systemic findings of high fevers, chills, and marked toxicity are often present. Progression of the infection may lead to respiratory obstruction, septicemia, and osteomyelitis of the adjacent facial bones.

The predominant bacterial pathogen is *S. aureus*. However, streptococci (including *S. pneumoniae)* and anaerobes (primarily *Bacteroides* sp., *Peptostreptococcus* sp., and *Prevotella* sp.) may also play an important role. Aerobic gram-negative bacteria (e.g., *E. coli)* may also cause acute parotitis, particularly in hospitalized patients. Other less common organisms include *E. corrodens, Arachnia, H. influenzae, T. pallidum,* cat-scratch bacillus, *M. tuberculosis,* and atypical mycobacteria. Early appropriate antimicrobial therapy may prevent suppuration. Initial empiric therapy should cover common pathogens, including *S. aureus,* and anaerobes (e.g., cefazolin,

**229**

penicillinase-resistant penicillin, and clindamycin). Maintenance of adequate hydration is essential. Although most patients with acute parotitis respond to antimicrobial therapy, surgical intervention is occasionally indicated for drainage of abscesses.

## SUGGESTED READINGS

Brook I: Diagnosis and management of parotitis, *Arch Otolaryngol Head Neck Surg* 118:469-471, 1992.

Brook I, Frazier EH, Thompson DH: Aerobic and anaerobic microbiology of acute suppurative parotitis, *Laryngoscope* 101:170-172, 1991.

Chow AW: Infections of the oral cavity, neck, and head. In Mandell GL, Bennett JE, Dolin R, eds: *Principles and practices of infectious diseases,* ed 4, New York, 1995, Churchill Livingstone.

# Penicillin Allergy

Q  Is it safe to use cephalosporins in a patient with penicillin allergy?

Patients with a history of penicillin allergy have been reported to have allergic reactions to cephalosporins at a rate of 5% to 16.5% compared with 1% to 2.5% for patients with a negative history of penicillin allergy. However, these rates are based on studies with several problems. First, a positive history of penicillin allergy is not reliable in the majority of patients (60% to 85%) based on results of negative penicillin skin testing in persons reporting such allergy. Second, many of the reactions reported as allergic response to cephalosporins were likely not immune mediated. Finally, persons with a history of penicillin allergy are 3 times more likely to have adverse reactions to other drugs, including those not related to penicillin; therefore allergy to cephalosporins in these patients may not necessarily reflect immunological cross-reactivity with penicillin.

Immunological cross-reactivity with penicillin appears to be more common with first-generation cephalosporins (e.g., cefazolin) and less common with third-generation cephalosporins. For example, the relative risk of allergic reaction to ceftazidime in those with penicillin allergy is 1.6 compared with 4 for first- and second-generation cephalosporins.

In general, a history of anaphylactic reaction to penicillin (type I hypersensitivity reaction) should lead to avoidance of cephalosporins. In contrast, when penicillin reaction is less severe (e.g., fever, eosinophilia, or rash), cephalosporins may be administered cautiously.

SUGGESTED READINGS

Lin RY: A perspective on penicillin allergy, *Arch Intern Med* 152:930-937, 1992.
Saxon A et al: Immediate hypersensitivity reactions to beta-lactam antibiotics [clinical conference], *Ann Intern Med* 107:204-215, 1987.
Sher TH: Penicillin hypersensitivity: a review, *Pediatr Clin North Am* 30:161-176, 1983.

 Can imipenem/cilastatin (Primaxin) be used safely in patients with penicillin allergy?

Imipenem is a synthetic congener of thienamycin, a carbapenem antibiotic with a beta-lactam ring. Patients who demonstrate IgE-mediated response to minor penicillin determinants appear to also demonstrate a high degree of immunological cross-reactivity to the analogous imipenem determinants. Therefore this antibiotic should not be administered to those patients with immediate hypersensitivity reaction to penicillin without the same precaution necessary when administering penicillin to such patients.

SUGGESTED READINGS

Adelman DC: New beta-lactam antibiotics. In Saxon A, moderator: Immediate hypersensitivity reactions to beta-lactam antibiotics, *Ann Intern Med* 107:204-215, 1987.
Lipman B, Neu HC: Imipenem: a new carbapenem antibiotic, *Med Clin North Am* 72:567-579, 1988.

Can aztreonam (Azactam) be administered safely to patients with penicillin allergy?

Aztreonam is a monobactam, a novel group of beta-lactam antibiotics. To date, there are no data to suggest immunological cross-reactivity between penicillins and aztreonam. Even patients with IgE antibodies to penicillin determinants appear to have no allergic reaction to aztreonam. Thus aztreonam may be safely administered to patients with penicillin allergy.

SUGGESTED READING

Adelman DC: New beta-lactam antibiotics. In Saxon A, moderator: Immediate hypersensitivity reactions to beta-lactam antibiotics, *Ann Intern Med* 107:204-215, 1987.

Enterococcal UTI has been diagnosed in a patient with penicillin allergy. What alternative antibiotics besides ampicillin can be used?

Nitrofurantoin (Macrodantin) may be considered in patients *without* pyelonephritis, prostatic infection, bacteremia, or renal insufficiency (creatinine clearance less than 40 ml/min). In vitro, nitrofurantoin is active against more than 90% of *E. faecalis* strains but only 50% of *E. faecium* isolates. The usual dose of nitrofurantoin is 50 to 100 mg 4×/day PO; no parenteral form is available. For prophylaxis of recurrent UTIs, 50 to 100 mg/day is commonly recommended.

Quinolones (e.g., ciprofloxacin) may also be considered for UTIs caused by enterococci, but many strains are becoming resistant to these antibiotics.

Vancomycin may also be considered if the enterococcal isolate is susceptible in vitro to this drug. Oral form of vancomycin is poorly absorbed and therefore should *not* be used for treatment of systemic infections or UTIs.

## SUGGESTED READINGS

Fekety R: Vancomycin and teicoplanin. In Mandell GL, Bennett JE, Dolin R, eds: *Principles and practices of infectious diseases,* ed 4, New York, 1995, Churchill Livingstone.

Hooper DC: Urinary tract agents: nitrofurantoin and methenamine. In Mandell GL, Bennett JE, Dolin R, eds: *Principles and practices of infectious diseases,* ed 4, New York, 1995, Churchill Livingstone.

 How is a patient with syphilis and penicillin allergy treated?*

For primary or secondary syphilis, doxycycline 100 mg PO 2×/day for 14 days, tetracycline hydrochloride 500 mg PO 4×/day for 14 days, ceftriaxone (1 g IM every 2 days for four doses or 250 mg daily for 10 days or 500 mg every 2 days for five doses), or azithromycin 500 mg daily for 10 days may be effective.

---

*Only 10% of persons who report a history of severe allergic reactions to penicillin are still allergic. Skin testing with the major and minor determinants is useful in identifying persons at high risk for penicillin reactions. Patients who report a history of penicillin reaction and are skin-test negative by the full battery of penicillin reagents (major and minor determinants) can receive conventional penicillin therapy. Persons who have a positive skin test to one of the penicillin determinants can be desensitized. PO desensitization is considered to be safer and simpler than IV. Patients should be desensitized in a hospital setting because of risk of serious IgE-mediated allergic reactions. A schedule of oral penicillin desensitization is found in the Centers for Disease Control and Prevention *MMWR* supplement listed in the references for this section.

For latent syphilis, doxycycline or tetracycline for 2 weeks at previously mentioned doses is recommended if duration of infection is known to have been less than 1 year; otherwise, for 4 weeks. Ceftriaxone 1 to 2 g IV or IM once daily for 10 to 14 days is moderately effective in HIV-infected patients with latent syphilis or neurosyphilis.

For neurosyphilis, penicillin desensitization or ceftriaxone should be considered. Input from an infectious diseases expert is recommended.

Note:  1.  *Penicillin allergy should be documented before choosing alternative therapy.*
2.  *Because therapeutic regimens other than penicillin have usually not been well studied, careful follow-up is mandatory.*
3.  *Pregnant women with syphilis and penicillin allergy should undergo penicillin allergy skin testing and desensitization if necessary. Tetracyclines are contraindicated during pregnancy.*

## SUGGESTED READINGS

Centers for Disease Control and Prevention: 1993 sexually transmitted diseases treatment guidelines, *MMWR* 42(RR-14):1-102, 1993.

Dowell ME et al: Response of latent syphilis or neurosyphilis to ceftriaxone therapy in persons infected with human immunodeficiency, *Am J Med* 93:477-479, 1992.

Hook EW III, Roddy RE, Handsfield HH: Ceftriaxone therapy for incubating and early syphilis, *J Infect Dis* 158:881-884, 1988.

Schofer H, Vogt HJ, Milbradt R: Ceftriaxone for the treatment of primary and secondary syphilis, *Chemotherapy* 35:140-145, 1989.

Verdon MS, Handsfield HH, Johnson RB: Pilot study of azithromycin for treatment of primary and secondary syphilis, *Clin Infect Dis* 19:486-488, 1994.

# Peritonitis

Q
What is the appropriate management of spontaneous bacterial peritonitis (SBP)?

Antibiotic coverage should be directed against the most likely pathogens causing SBP: aerobic bacteria of the normal intestinal flora. Together, *E. coli* (approximately 50%), *Klebsiella* sp. (approximately 10%), and streptococci (approximately 30%) account for nearly 90% of cases of SBP; anaerobic infection is rare (presumably because of the high oxygen tension of ascitic fluid) and should suggest secondary peritonitis caused by perforated viscus. The great majority (over 90%) of SBPs are related to a single organism. Third-generation cephalosporins (e.g., cefotaxime 2 g IV every 8 hrs; ceftriaxone 2 g IV every 24 hrs) are considered the drugs of choice, because they cover enteric aerobic gram-negative bacilli and many streptococci. Ticarcillin/clavulanate and piperacillin-tazobactam should also be effective.

Aztreonam should *not* be used as initial monotherapy of SBP because of the relatively higher risk of superinfection secondary to gram-positive organisms. Similarly, aminoglycosides should *not* generally be used because of the risk of nephrotoxicity and suboptimal response.

Following initiation of appropriate antibiotic(s), repeat paracentesis at 48 hours is recommended to document decreasing number of polymorphonuclear (PMN) cells. If PMN count is less than 250/ml at that time, a 5- to 7-day course of antibi-

**236**

otic therapy should be sufficient. A repeat paracentesis after completion of therapy is not routinely recommended. Conversely, if the PMN count is greater than baseline values or culture of ascites remains positive, either drug resistance or secondary peritonitis should be considered.

## SUGGESTED READINGS

Bhuva M, Ganger D, Jensen D: Spontaneous bacterial peritonitis: an update on evaluation, management, and prevention, *Am J Med* 97:169-175, 1994.

Gilbert JA, Kamath PS: Spontaneous bacterial peritonitis: an update, *Mayo Clin Proc* 70:365-370, 1995.

Hoefs JC: Spontaneous bacterial peritonitis: prevention and therapy, *Hepatology* 12:776-781, 1990.

 What is the role of antibiotic therapy in prevention of SBP?

Because of the high recurrence rates associated with SBP (approximately 70% at 1 year), antibiotic prophylaxis against this condition has been attempted. Two relatively well-tolerated oral antibiotics that have been shown to significantly reduce the frequency of SBPs in patients with ascites at high risk of SBP include norfloxacin (400 mg/day) and trimethoprim-sulfamethoxazole (double-strength tablet 5×/week, Monday through Friday). However, antibiotic prophylaxis may not reduce mortality or the number of readmissions to the hospital. The cost-effectiveness of long-term antibiotic prophylaxis has not yet been established. Short-term antibiotic prophylaxis has been advocated in patients admitted to the hospital with gastrointestinal hemorrhage or acute liver failure because these patients are least likely to survive an episode of SBP.

## SUGGESTED READINGS

Bhuva M, Ganger D, Jensen D: Spontaneous bacterial peritonitis: an update on evaluation, management, and prevention, *Am J Med* 97:169-75, 1994.

Gilbert JA, Kamath PS: Spontaneous bacterial peritonitis: an update, *Mayo Clin Proc* 70:365-370, 1995.

Singh N et al: Trimethoprim-sulfamethoxazole for the prevention of spontaneous bacterial peritonitis in cirrhosis: a randomized trial, *Ann Intern Med* 122:595-598, 1995.

# Pharyngitis

 What are the causes of pharyngitis?

Pharyngitis is an inflammatory syndrome of the oropharynx primarily associated with infectious causes but also occasionally associated with noninfectious processes.

Viral causes account for the majority of pharyngitis cases and include rhinoviruses, enteroviruses, adenoviruses, influenza and parainfluenza viruses, EBV, and herpes simplex virus.

Bacterial causes include *Streptococcus pyogenes* (accounting for approximately 10% of pharyngitis in adults and as high as 40% to 50% in children and adolescents), *Chlamydia trachomatis* (found in up to 20% of patients with pharyngitis accompanied by respiratory symptoms), *M. pneumoniae* (associated with 11% of pharyngitis in adults and as high as 32% in children), *N. gonorrhoeae, Corynebacterium haemolyticum, C. diphtheriae, M. tuberculosis, Francisella tularensis,* and mixed anaerobes (Vincent's angina). Toxic shock and Kawasaki syndromes are also often associated with pharyngitis.

*C. albicans* may cause pharyngitis in immunocompromised patients or those on steroids or antibiotics.

Noninfectious causes of pharyngitis include injuries, malignancy, aphthous ulcers (e.g., Behçet's syndrome and canker sores), pemphigus vulgaris, chemotherapy-induced mucositis, and allergic reactions (e.g., Stevens-Johnson syndrome).

**239**

SUGGESTED READINGS

Todd JK: The sore throat: pharyngitis and epiglottitis, *Infect Dis Clin North Am* 2:149-162, 1988.

Vukmir RB: Adult and pediatric pharyngitis: a review, *J Emerg Med* 10:607-616, 1992.

*Q* How should patients who have treatment failure or relapse after penicillin therapy for group A streptococcal pharyngitis be managed?

Such individuals may benefit from treatment with an antibiotic that is not inactivated by oropharyngeal penicillinase-producing organisms (e.g., amoxicillin/clavulanate acid, cloxacillin, dicloxacillin, erythromycin, clindamycin, or rifampin given concurrently during the last 4 days of the 10-day regimen of oral penicillin). Clindamycin has been shown to be effective in eradicating chronic group A streptococci pharyngeal carriage. The following antibiotics should *not* be used for treatment of group A streptococcal pharyngitis: tetracyclines, sulfonamides, trimethoprim, and chloramphenicol.

SUGGESTED READINGS

Bass JW: Antibiotic management of group A streptococcal pharyngotonsillitis, *Pediatr Infect Dis* 10(suppl 10):S43-S49, 1991.

Peter G: Streptococcal pharyngitis: current therapy and criteria for evaluation of new agents, *Clin Infect Dis* 14(suppl 2):S218-S223, 1992.

How should patients with throat cultures growing group C or G beta-hemolytic streptococci be managed? Can these organisms cause pharyngitis?

Both group C and G streptococci may colonize human pharynx without causing any symptoms (1% to 2% colonization rates in adults). However, these streptococci have also been associated with outbreaks of pharyngitis, including those related to ingestion of contaminated animal products (e.g., eggs, milk, and cheese). Moreover, in recent years there has been mounting evidence that groups C and G streptococci may be associated with endemic or sporadically acquired pharyngitis. The clinical symptoms and course may be similar to that of group A streptococcal pharyngitis (e.g., fever, mild to severe sore throat, pharyngeal exudates, and cervical lymphadenopathy). In contrast to group A *Streptococcus*, these organisms are not associated with the development of rheumatic fever; post-streptococcal glomerulonephritis following group C streptococcal pharyngitis has been reported, however.

Additional considerations include the following:

1.   Because of the similarities between streptolysin O produced by group G and certain group C streptococci *(S. equisimilis)* and group A *Streptococcus*, infections caused by these organisms may also be associated with a rise in serum anti-streptolysin O (ASO) titers.

2.   Commercially available rapid throat swab streptococcal tests are specific only for group A *Streptococcus* and therefore may not detect the presence of groups C and G streptococci.

3.   Penicillin G, first-generation cephalosporins, and vancomycin have good in vitro activity against groups C and G

streptococci. Erythromycin and tetracyclines have variable in vitro activity against group C streptococci. Clindamycin, erythromycin, and chloramphenicol have relatively poor bactericidal activity against group G streptococci. Although the optimal therapy for pharyngitis caused by these organisms is unclear, treatment with an in vitro active oral agent—similar to the regimen used for group A *Streptococcus*—may be considered.

## SUGGESTED READINGS

Cimolai N et al: Do the beta-hemolytic non-group A streptococci cause pharyngitis? *Rev Infect Dis* 10:587-601, 1988.

Gerber MA et al: Community-wide outbreak of group G streptococcal pharyngitis, *Pediatrics* 87:598-603, 1991.

Johnson CC, Tunkel AR: Viridans streptococci and groups C and G streptococci. In Mandell GL, Bennett JE, Dolin R, eds: *Principles and practices of infectious diseases,* ed 4, New York, 1995, Churchill Livingstone.

Turner JC et al: Role of group C beta-hemolytic streptococci in pharyngitis: epidemiologic study of clinical features associated with isolation of group C streptococci, *J Clin Microbiol* 31:808-811, 1993.

Vukmir RB: Adult and pediatric pharyngitis: a review, *J Emerg Med* 10:607-616, 1992.

## STIMULATING QUESTION

Is *H. influenzae* a cause of pharyngitis?

Although *H. influenzae* may cause a variety of respiratory tract infections such as pneumonia, epiglottitis, and sinusitis, its etiological role as a primary cause of pharyngitis is weak at best. Indeed, this organism is not even listed as a cause of pharyngitis in a major infectious disease textbook (in the following reference list).

## SUGGESTED READINGS

Gwaltney JM: Pharyngitis. In Mandell GL, Bennett JE, Dolin R, eds: *Principles and practices of infectious diseases,* ed 4, New York, 1995, Churchill Livingstone.

Todd JK: The sore throat: pharyngitis and epiglottitis, *Infect Dis Clin North Am* 2:149-162, 1988.

# Prosthetic Joints

Should patients with prosthetic joints receive antibiotic prophylaxis similar to that used for endocarditis prophylaxis when undergoing dental procedures?

Although the majority of orthopedists and dentists recommend antibiotic prophylaxis before patients with prosthetic joints undergo dental procedures likely to cause a transient bacteremia, this practice appears to be based more on myth and fear of litigation than scientific facts.

The facts include the following:

1. There are significant differences between late prosthetic valve endocarditis and late prosthetic joint infection (e.g., oral streptococci are infrequently a cause of late prosthetic joint infection, whereas they account for up to 25% of late prosthetic valve infections).

2. There are few cases of late prosthetic joint infection after dental treatment, and the association between the latter and septic arthritis is at best weak; most cases of prosthetic joint infections are not caused by dental procedures.

3. Animal experiments have not demonstrated a cause-and-effect relationship between dental procedures and late prosthetic joint infections.

4. The risks and costs of antibiotic prophylaxis for dental procedures in patients with prosthetic joints appear to outweigh the potential benefits; the mortality from late infection caused by transient bacteremia may be similar to the estimated number of deaths from anaphylactic reaction to the antibiotic.

Some authors have recommended antibiotic prophylaxis before dental procedures only in selected patients who seem to be at high risk of late prosthetic joint infection: patients with rheumatoid arthritis; diabetes mellitus; reoperated, loosened, or previously infected joints, particularly hips; and immunosuppression (e.g., those on steroids) who are undergoing procedures for greater than 3 minutes that are likely to be associated with bacteremia.

In summary, there is no convincing evidence to support routine antibiotic prophylaxis before dental procedures for patients with prosthetic joints. At the most, selected patients at high risk of late prosthetic joint infection may be considered for antibiotic prophylaxis, but scientific evidence of the efficacy of this practice in preventing prosthetic joint infections is also lacking.

Note: *Regardless of the uncertainties of the efficacy of antibiotic prophylaxis, it is essential to aggressively treat all dental and cutaneous infections in patients with prosthetic joints.*

### SUGGESTED READINGS

Averns HL, Kerry R: Role of prophylactic antibiotics in the prevention of late infection of prosthetic joints. Results of a questionnaire and review of the literature, *Br J Rheum* 34:380-382, 1995.

Jacobson JJ, Schweitzer SO, Kowalski CJ: Chemoprophylaxis of prosthetic joint patients during dental treatment: a decision-utility analysis, *Oral Surg Oral Med Oral Pathol* 72:167-177, 1991.

Manian FA: Prosthetic joint infection due to *Haemophilus parainfluenzae* after dental surgery [letter], *South Med J* 84:807-808, 1991.

Thyne GM, Ferguson JW: Antibiotic prophylaxis during dental treatment in patients with prosthetic joints, *J Bone Joint Surg [Br]* 73-B:191-194, 1991.

Wahl MJ: Myths of dental-induced prosthetic joint infections, *Clin Infect Dis* 20:1420-1425, 1995.

# Rheumatic Fever

How should acute rheumatic fever be diagnosed?

The 1992 updated Jones criteria for the diagnosis of initial attack of rheumatic fever requires *the presence of two major manifestations or one major and two minor manifestations, in the presence of evidence of preceding group A streptococcal infection* (i.e., microbiologically documented streptococcal pharyngitis, a positive throat culture or rapid antigen test for group A streptococci, or the demonstration of an elevated or rising streptococcal antibody titer).

## MAJOR MANIFESTATIONS

Carditis
Polyarthritis
Chorea
Erythema marginatum
Subcutaneous nodules

## MINOR MANIFESTATIONS

Arthralgia
Fever
Elevated erythrocyte sedimentation rate (ESR) or C-reactive protein
Prolonged PR interval

**247**

## ADDITIONAL CONSIDERATIONS

1. Failure to fulfill the above criteria makes the diagnosis of acute rheumatic fever unlikely except in three situations: Sydenham's chorea, indolent carditis, and in case of a recurrent attack in a patient with previously documented rheumatic fever (e.g., in a patient with known rheumatic heart disease in whom diagnosis of acute carditis may be difficult unless a different valve is involved).

2. Evidence of recent streptococcal infection is an integral part of the revised Jones criteria.

3. Group A streptococcal skin infections do not give rise to acute rheumatic fever.

4. Clinical history of sore throat or of scarlet fever not confirmed by laboratory data is not adequate evidence of recent group A streptococcal infection.

SUGGESTED READINGS

Anonymous: Guidelines for the diagnosis of rheumatic fever: Jones criteria, *JAMA* 268:2069-2073, 1992.
Bisno AL: Nonsuppurative poststreptococcal sequelae: rheumatic fever and glomerulonephritis. In Mandell GL, Bennett JE, Dolin R, eds: *Principles and practices of infectious diseases,* ed 4, New York, 1995, Churchill Livingstone.

 What are some explanations for an elevated ASO titer?

Beta-hemolytic streptococci belonging to group A, C, or G produce an enzyme known as *streptolysin O.* About 7 to 10 days after infection with these organisms, ASO antibodies may appear. The highest incidence of reactivity is during the third week following onset of acute rheumatic fever, with 80% to

85% of patients having abnormal results at this time. There-after, the antibody titer falls steadily: 70% to 75% positive results at 2 months; 35% at 6 months; and 20% at 12 months. Consequently, an abnormal ASO titer (usually greater than 200 Todd units) may suggest recent streptococcal infection.

*A positive ASO titer is not by itself diagnostic of acute rheumatic fever.* Several situations and conditions may be associated with elevated ASO titers without evidence of concurrent rheumatic fever, including rheumatoid arthritis, postinfec-tious arthritis, psoriatic arthritis, ankylosing spondylitis, sar-coidosis, Still's disease, vasculitis, septic arthritis, and arthral-gia/myalgia associated with HLA-B27 positivity. An elevated ASO titer without rheumatic fever may also be found in some healthy persons, those with ischemic heart disease, and those with a relatively distant streptococcal infection with slowly declining ASO titers.

The pathogenesis of reactive arthritis following streptococcal infection may be caused by the shared epitope between the surface M protein of streptococci and antigens of articular cartilage and synovium leading to tissue injury mediated by cross-reactive antibodies. Thus reactive arthritis may be asso-ciated with evidence of recent streptococcal infection and elevated ASO titers, without meeting the Jones criteria for rheumatic fever.

## SUGGESTED READINGS

Eichbaum QG et al: Rheumatic fever: autoantibodies against a variety of cardiac, nuclear, and streptococcal antigens, *Ann Rheum Dis* 54:740-743, 1995.

Ravel R: *Clinical laboratory medicine: clinical application of laboratory data,* ed 6, St Louis, 1995, Mosby.

Schattner A: Poststreptococcal reactive rheumatic syndrome, *J Rheumatol* 23:1297-1298, 1996.

Valtonen JM et al: Various rheumatic syndromes in adult patients associ-ated with high antistreptolysin O titers and their differential diagnosis with rheumatic fever, *Ann Rheum Dis* 52:527-530, 1993.

When can antibiotic prophylaxis against rheumatic fever be safely discontinued?

The optimal duration of continuous antimicrobial prophylaxis (e.g., benzathine penicillin G 1.2 million U IM every 4 weeks, penicillin V 250 mg or erythromycin 250 mg 2 ×/day) remains unclear and should be individualized. Although some authorities have recommended lifelong prophylaxis in patients with established bouts of rheumatic fever, given the decline in the incidence of this condition with age and with the number of years following the most recent attack, some patients may be able to safely discontinue prophylaxis.

The risk of recurrence appears to be quite low in older adults without heart disease who are not in intimate contact with school-age children; under these circumstances, prophylaxis may be discontinued after 5 years or at age 18, whichever is longer, as long as the patient is carefully monitored. Similarly, in patients with only mild mitral regurgitation or healed carditis, discontinuation of prophylaxis after 10 years or at age 25, whichever is longer, has been suggested. Until further data become available, those with aortic valvular disease, mitral stenosis, or polyvalvular involvement should receive prophylaxis for life.

## POINTS TO REMEMBER

1. Symptomatic intercurrent streptococcal throat infections should be treated with an appropriate antibiotic.

2. Patients with residual rheumatic valvular disease should receive additional antibiotic prophylaxis against bacterial endocarditis whenever they undergo dental or invasive pro-

cedures that consistently cause bacteremia or are known to be associated with the development of endocarditis.

SUGGESTED READINGS

Berrios X et al: Discontinuing rheumatic fever prophylaxis in selected adolescents and young adults: a prospective study, *Ann Intern Med* 118:401-406, 1993.

Bisno AL: Nonsuppurative poststreptococcal sequelae: rheumatic fever and glomerulonephritis. In Mandell GL, Bennett JE, Dolin R, eds: *Principles and practices of infectious diseases,* ed 4, New York, 1995, Churchill Livingstone.

# Sinusitis

 How should community-acquired acute sinusitis be managed?

Although viruses may play a role in the pathogenesis of acute sinusitis (defined as infection in a paranasal sinus lasting from 1 day to 3 weeks), the disease is treated as a bacterial infection. The mainstay of therapy is empiric use of antibacterial agents (commonly oral and as outpatient) and supportive therapy. In certain cases, otolaryngological consultation should also be considered (see the following section).

## ANTIMICROBIAL THERAPY

In adults, acute community-acquired sinusitis is most commonly caused by *H. influenzae* or *S. pneumoniae*. Anaerobic bacteria may play a role in patients with dental disease. *S. aureus, S. pyogenes, M. catarrhalis,* and alpha-hemolytic and other streptococci may also play a role in acute sinusitis. *S. aureus* is the major pathogen in acute sphenoid and frontal sinusitis. *C. pneumoniae* has also been implicated, but given the frequent response of acute sinusitis to antibiotics that are not active against this agent, its overall importance in the causation of community-acquired sinusitis remains unclear.

Timely antibiotic coverage against the common bacterial sinusitis is important for prevention of complications and avoidance of development of chronic sinusitis. Antibiotic therapy is usually empiric because of the lack of correlation between the organisms identified on nasopharyngeal culture and those isolated from sinus aspiration. Trimethoprim-sulfamethoxazole (160 mg/800 mg, 2×/day), amoxicillin/clavulanate (500 mg/125 mg 3×/day), cefuroxime axetil (250 mg 2×/day), cefixime (400 mg 1×/day), azithromycin (500 mg initial dose, followed by 250 mg 1×/day), and clarithromycin (500 mg 2×/day) are effective treatment for most cases of acute sinusitis. Amoxicillin and ampicillin are no longer recommended as first-line agents because of the widespread prevalence of beta-lactamase–producing organisms (e.g., *H. influenzae* and *M. catarrhalis)* causing acute sinusitis. Similarly, penicillin, first-generation cephalosporins, or tetracyclines should not be used as a first-line agent.

Duration of therapy is typically for 10 to 14 days, although a 3-day course of trimethoprim-sulfamethoxazole may also be effective. For azithromycin, a 5-day course has been shown to be effective.

In the small percentage (10% or less) of patients who do not show adequate response to initial therapy with a beta-lactam antibiotic or trimethoprim-sulfamethoxazole, treatment for *C. pneumoniae* with tetracycline, erythromycin, or a newer macrolide (e.g., clarithromycin or azithromycin) is reasonable.

In patients with HIV infection, *P. aeruginosa* may also be an important cause of acute sinusitis. Treatment with an appropriate antipseudomonal antibiotic (e.g., ciprofloxacin, ceftazidime, ticarcillin, piperacillin, or gentamicin) selected based on in vitro susceptibility test results is necessary. Similarly, in diabetics with ketoacidosis and in neutropenic patients, coverage for gram-negative bacteria and opportunistic fungi needs to be considered.

## SUPPORTIVE THERAPY

Adjunctive therapies such as oral and topical decongestants and mucolytics (e.g., guaifenesin) are commonly recommended. Antihistamines are relatively contraindicated in patients with acute sinusitis because of concerns over drying of mucous membranes and interference with the clearing of secretions.

## OTOLARYNGOLOGICAL CONSULTATION

Referral to an otolaryngologist should be considered when there is a need for nasal endoscopy, diagnostic antral puncture to obtain material for culture, or therapeutic irrigation. Specifically, complicated sinusitis with extension of infection into the orbits or cranium, frontal or sphenoid sinusitis, deterioration within 2 days, treatment failure after two courses of appropriate antibiotics, and frequent recurrences (more than three bouts of acute sinusitis per year) should prompt consultation with an otolaryngologist.

### SUGGESTED READINGS

Diaz I, Bamberger DM: Acute sinusitis, *Semin Resp Infect* 10:14-20, 1995.

Gwaltney JM: Sinusitis. In Mandell GL, Bennett JE, Dolin R, eds: *Principles and practices of infectious diseases,* ed 4, New York, 1995, Churchill Livingstone.

O'Donnell JG et al: Sinusitis due to *Pseudomonas aeruginosa* in patients with human immunodeficiency virus infection, *Clin Infect Dis* 16:404-406, 1993.

Reuler JB, Lucas LM, Kumar KL: Sinusitis: a review for generalists, *West J Med* 163:40-48, 1995.

Williams JW Jr et al: Randomized controlled trial of 3 vs 10 days of trimethoprim/sulfamethoxazole for acute maxillary sinusitis, *JAMA* 273:1015-1021, 1995.

How should chronic sinusitis be managed?

When symptoms of sinusitis (e.g., purulent nasal discharge, nasal obstruction, facial pain, headaches, chronic cough, and halitosis) persist longer than 3 months, chronic sinusitis may be diagnosed. As opposed to the acute and subacute stages (3 weeks to 3 months), the epithelial damage in the sinus is not usually reversible, and impairment of drainage of the sinus cavity is the rule. Thus even though bacterial colonization of the sinus cavity is common in chronic sinusitis, this condition is usually considered a disease of mucosal damage rather than an infectious state. Surgical intervention, particularly endoscopic sinus surgery, is often needed to facilitate sinus drainage.

Acute infectious exacerbations of chronic sinusitis should be managed similarly to acute sinusitis, but a longer course of antibiotic therapy (3 weeks or more) may be necessary. Some authors recommend treatment with antibiotics with in vitro activity against anaerobes (e.g., amoxicillin/clavulanate, clindamycin, or metronidazole); recent studies, however, have shown a relatively low rate (<10%) of isolation of anaerobes in chronic sinusitis. Control of allergies is important.

## SUGGESTED READINGS

Gwaltney JM: Sinusitis. In Mandell GL, Bennett JE, Dolin R, eds: *Principles and practices of infectious diseases,* ed 4, New York, 1995, Churchill Livingstone.

Mabry RL: Therapeutic agents in the medical management of sinusitis, *Otolaryngol Clin North Am* 26:561-570, 1993.

Ramadan HH: What is the bacteriology of chronic sinusitis in adults? *Am J Otolaryngol* 16:303-306, 1995.

Reuler JB, Lucas LM, Kumar KL: Sinusitis: a review for generalists, *West J Med* 163:40-48, 1995.

How often is nosocomial sinusitis a cause of fever in hospitalized patients, and how should it be managed?

From 15% to 20% of radiographically diagnosed sinusitis in critically ill patients may be associated with fever or signs of sepsis. Nosocomial sinusitis may also be associated with nosocomial lower respiratory tract infection, with the sinuses possibly serving as a reservoir of potential pathogens for the lower respiratory tract.

Removal of potential risk factors for nosocomial sinusitis is an important part of its treatment; these include nasogastric tube, nasotracheal tube, and nasal packing. Otolaryngological consultation should be considered for diagnostic sinus aspiration for cultures and antrum lavage. Antimicrobial therapy should be based on sinus aspirate gram stain and cultures. Common isolates from nosocomially infected sinus cavities include aerobic gram-negative bacteria (e.g., *P. aeruginosa, Enterobacteriaceae,* and *Acinetobacter*), *S. aureus,* and at times yeast (18% in one study). While waiting for cultures, empiric use of antipseudomonal antibiotics such as ticarcillin/clavulanate, piperacillin-tazobactam, or ceftazidime, in combination with an aminoglycoside, is reasonable.

### SUGGESTED READINGS

Borman KR et al: Occult fever in surgical intensive care unit patients is seldom caused by sinusitis, *Am J Surg* 164:412-416, 1992.

Lum Cheong RS, Cornwell EE III: Suppurative sinusitis in critically ill patients: a case report and review of the literature, *J Natl Med Assoc* 84:1057-1059, 1992.

Reuler JB, Lucas LM, Kumar KL: Sinusitis: a review for generalists, *West J Med* 163:40-48, 1995.

Rouby JJ et al: Risk factors and clinical relevance of nosocomial maxillary sinusitis in the critically ill, *Am J Resp Crit Care Med* 150:776-783, 1994.

My patient has *Aspergillus* sp. growing from his maxillary sinus aspirate. Is this significant? How should it be managed?

When faced with a patient with *Aspergillus* growth from the sinus aspirate, invasive (invading mucosal lining of the sinus wall or beyond) and noninvasive disease must be differentiated histologically before an appropriate course of treatment can be planned.

Invasive disease may be fulminant (acute) or indolent (chronic). It is characterized by spread of fungal mycelium from sinus air spaces into adjacent structures with tissue necrosis, chronic inflammation, and fibrosis. Invasion of blood vessels with resultant thrombosis and infarction is usually associated with the presence of fungal elements within the submucosa or bone. Fulminant aspergillosis of the sinuses occurs usually in neutropenic patients with lymphoreticular or hemopoietic malignancies and in bone marrow transplant patients. Indolent disease occurs in diabetic or AIDS patients and occasionally in immunologically normal patients; in the latter case, a granulomatous response is characteristic. Radiological investigations, including CT scan, should be performed to assess the extent of spread to the sinus wall, if any.

Treatment of invasive *Aspergillus* sinusitis should consist of surgical removal of all involved tissue in conjunction with antifungal therapy. Amphotericin B is the antifungal drug of choice in aspergillosis. The amphotericin B/lipid complex may be administered with less associated toxicity, but its high cost is likely to limit its use to those patients who are unresponsive to or unable to tolerate the nephrotoxicity of conventional amphotericin B. Itraconazole is a relatively non-toxic antifungal oral agent with efficacy against aspergillosis and may be used either singly (in relatively stable patients) or in combination with amphotericin B. Close clinical monitoring for evidence of recurrence of disease with follow-up CT scans is essential. Expert advice regarding management of this disease is recommended.

Noninvasive *Aspergillus* sinusitis may present in two forms: (1) localized with tangled fungal mycelium (aspergilloma) usually affecting a single sinus and often associated with chronic sinusitis and (2) allergic sinusitis occurring as a spectrum of disease ranging from mild sinus disease and atopy to severe sinusitis associated with extremely high total IgE levels, not unlike allergic bronchopulmonary aspergillosis. Treatment should be aimed at surgical removal of fungal elements and inflamed tissue, which may be curative by itself. In allergic *Aspergillus* sinusitis, postoperative use of topical intranasal steroids should be considered. Although treatment with systemic corticosteroids has been advocated by some authors as adjunctive therapy for *Aspergillus* sinusitis, its role remains controversial; it may be considered, however, in recurrent disease and in the setting of severe atopy. *Use of antifungal agents is not recommended for treatment of allergic* Aspergillus *sinusitis without invasive disease.* Long-term follow-up of patients for recurrent disease is recommended.

### SUGGESTED READINGS

Allphin AL, Strauss M, Abdul-Karim FW: Allergic fungal sinusitis: problems in diagnosis and treatment, *Laryngoscope* 101:815-820, 1991.
de Carpentier JP et al: An algorithmic approach to *Aspergillus* sinusitis, *J Laryngol Otol* 108:314-318, 1994.
Hartwick RW, Batsakis JG: Sinus aspergillosis and allergic fungal sinusitis, *Ann Otol Rhinol Laryngol* 100:427-430, 1991.

# Staphylococcus aureus

 How should teichoic acid (TA) antibody test results be interpreted?

TA is a structural component of gram-positive organisms. The TA serological assays detect antibodies against ribitol TA residues found primarily in *S. aureus,* as opposed to the glycerol residues found in other gram-positive bacteria. The commercially available assay for TA antibody (ENDO-STAPH) has a sensitivity of 60%, specificity of 85%, positive predictive value of 54%, and negative predictive value of 92% for metastatic septic complication following *S. aureus* bacteremia. A positive result is defined as a titer of 1:4 or greater or a fourfold or greater rise in titer.

The major role of the assay is in identification of patients in whom complications may develop following an episode of *S. aureus* bacteremia (e.g., intravascular device related) even though they seem to be doing well clinically. A positive titer after 2 weeks of therapy should raise suspicion for a sequestered focus of infection. Less commonly, TA antibody assay may be used in suspecting *S. aureus* as a cause of infection, which may be culture-negative because of prior antibiotic therapy (e.g., osteomyelitis). It should be noted that 3% of normal population may have a positive TA antibody. Therefore this test should only complement, not replace clinical judgment.

**259**

## SUGGESTED READINGS

Sheagren JN: Guidelines for the use of the teichoic acid antibody assay, *Arch Intern Med* 144:250-252, 1984.

Wheat J et al: Commercially available (ENDO-STAPH) assay for teichoic acid antibodies: evaluation in patients with serious *Staphylococcus aureus* infections and in controls, *Arch Intern Med* 144:261-264, 1984.

 Is trimethoprim-sulfamethoxazole active against *S. aureus?*

Trimethoprim-sulfamethoxazole has an excellent spectrum of activity against many *S. aureus* isolates, including those resistant to methicillin (MRSA). In IV drug users with methicillin-susceptible *S. aureus* infections (primarily tricuspid valve endocarditis), trimethoprim-sulfamethoxazole may not be as effective as vancomycin in eradication of infection; for methicillin-resistant isolates it appears to have similar efficacy.

## SUGGESTED READINGS

Markowitz N, Quinn EL, Saravolatz LD: Trimethoprim-sulfamethoxazole compared with vancomycin for the treatment of *Staphylococcus aureus* infection, *Ann Intern Med* 117:390-398, 1992.

Sheagren JN: *Staphylococcus aureus:* the persistent pathogen. II, *N Engl J Med* 22:1437-1442, 1984.

 Is ciprofloxacin active against *S. aureus?*

Although initial reports suggested good in vitro activity of ciprofloxacin against both methicillin-susceptible and methicillin-resistant *S. aureus* isolates, subsequent studies have demonstrated rapid emergence of resistance to this quinolone, particularly in those resistant to methicillin. Consequently, ciprofloxacin should not be used as primary therapy for *S. aureus* infections.

## SUGGESTED READINGS

Blumberg HM et al: Rapid development of ciprofloxacin resistance in methicillin-susceptible and -resistant *Staphylococcus aureus, J Infect Dis* 163:1279-1285, 1991.

Trucksis M, Hooper DC, Wolfson JS: Emerging resistance to fluoroquinolones in staphylococci: an alert, *Ann Intern Med* 114:424-425, 1991.

 How are serious infections caused by MRSA treated?

IV vancomycin is the drug of choice for treatment of serious MRSA infections (e.g., pneumonia, bacteremia, endocarditis, and wound infections). Rifampin is highly bactericidal for many strains of MRSA and may be useful when initial therapy with vancomycin is not successful or response to treatment is slow. Rifampin should never be used alone for treatment of MRSA infections because of emergence of resistance in this setting. Gentamicin may also be used in combination with vancomycin because of demonstrated in vitro synergy against most strains of MRSA with this combination even when the organisms are resistant to gentamicin; close monitoring for ototoxicity and nephrotoxicity is essential when these two drugs are used concurrently.

Trimethoprim-sulfamethoxazole has been effective in the treatment of MRSA endocarditis and bacteremia; however, in vitro susceptibility testing is recommended because of increasing number of resistant isolates. Minocycline has excellent in vitro activity against many MRSA strains and acts synergistically with rifampin in vitro.

Note: *The use of beta-lactams (e.g., penicillins and cephalosporins) and quinolones (e.g., ciprofloxacin) is not recommended for treatment of MRSA infections.*

### SUGGESTED READINGS

Markowitz N, Quinn EL, Saravolatz LD: Trimethoprim-sulfamethoxazole compared with vancomycin for the treatment of *Staphylococcus aureus* infection, *Ann Intern Med* 117:390-398, 1992.

Mulligan ME et al: Methicillin-resistant *Staphylococcus aureus:* a consensus review of the microbiology, pathogenesis, and epidemiology with implications for prevention and management, *Am J Med* 94:313-328, 1993.

When and how should MRSA colonization be eradicated?

Routine attempt at patient or staff MRSA decolonization is not advocated except under the following circumstances:

1. Colonized patients with relapsing MRSA infections

2. Colonized patients in the face of an ongoing outbreak despite other interventions

3. Colonized personnel epidemiologically associated with nosocomial outbreaks

Note: *Because of the relatively low risk of subsequent MRSA infection, patients should not undergo attempts at decolonization strictly for the purpose of transfer to a long-term care facility, and they should not be excluded from such facilities when colonized with MRSA.*

When MRSA nasal decolonization is indicated, the following regimens may be used:

1. 2% mupirocin ointment (Bactroban) to the nares 3×/day for 5 days

2. Trimethoprim-sulfamethoxazole (160 mg/800 mg or double-strength) PO every 12 hrs and rifampin 300 mg PO every 12 hrs for 7 days

3. Novobiocin 500 mg PO every 12 hrs and rifampin 300 mg PO every 12 hrs for 7 days

### SUGGESTED READINGS

Hartstein AI, Mulligan ME: Methicillin-resistant *Staphylococcus aureus.* In Mayhall CG, ed: *Hospital epidemiology and infection control,* Baltimore, 1996, Williams & Wilkins.

Mulligan ME et al: Methicillin-resistant *Staphylococcus aureus:* a consensus review of the microbiology, pathogenesis, and epidemiology with implications for prevention and management, *Am J Med* 94:313-328, 1993.

Walsh TJ et al: Randomized double-blinded trial of rifampin with either novobiocin or trimethoprim-sulfamethoxazole against methicillin-resistant *Staphylococcus aureus* colonization: prevention of antimicrobial resistance and effect of host factors on outcome, *Antimicrob Agents Chemother* 37:1334-1342, 1993.

 What isolation precautions do you recommend for patients with MRSA infection/colonization in health care facilities?

Policies aimed at the control of MRSA should take into account their impact on prevention of transmission from patient to patient, cost of patient care, and potential disruption of normal patient care activities in a given institution. As such, each institution should implement an infection

control policy that best serves the welfare of its patients without undue expense and unnecessary disruption of patient services. The following are general guidelines for isolation of MRSA culture-positive patients.

## COLONIZED/INFECTED HOSPITALIZED PATIENTS (E.G., RESPIRATORY TRACT, WOUND, AND BURNS)

Contact isolation: Standard/universal precautions in addition to private room or cohort with another infected/colonized patient, wearing gloves when entering the room and during the course of providing patient care, and washing hands following removal of gloves and before leaving the patient's room. Gowns are worn if substantial contact with the patient, environmental surfaces, or items in the patient's room is anticipated. Isolation is continued until the patient has discontinued antibiotics and is culture-negative.

## COLONIZED/INFECTED PATIENTS IN LONG-TERM CARE FACILITIES

Routine use of isolation and cohortation is not recommended except in the following circumstances for which contact isolation (outlined in previous section) should be considered: (1) outbreak setting; (2) patients with wounds heavily colonized by MRSA; and (3) patients with tracheostomies who are unable to handle secretions.

### SUGGESTED READINGS

Centers for Disease Control and Prevention: Guidelines for isolation precautions in hospitals, *Am J Infect Control* 24:24-52, 1996.

Mulligan ME et al: Methicillin-resistant *Staphylococcus aureus:* a consensus review of the microbiology, pathogenesis, and epidemiology with implications for prevention and management, *Am J Med* 94:313-328, 1993.

## STIMULATING QUESTION

What is the significance of a positive urine culture for *S. aureus* in patients with fever?

Primary UTIs caused by *S. aureus* are usually associated with the presence of urinary catheters. Secondary bacteremia from an initial urinary tract focus occurs in about 5% of patients with primary UTI from *S. aureus*. In patients without urinary catheters and *S. aureus* bacteriuria, a close search for a source of prior or current bacteremia (e.g., endocarditis) should be made.

### SUGGESTED READINGS

Lee BE, Crossley K, Gerding DN: The association between *Staphylococcus aureus* bacteremia and bacteriuria, *Am J Med* 65:303-306, 1978.

Sheagren JN: *Staphylococcus aureus:* the persistent pathogen. II, *N Engl J Med* 22:1437-1442, 1984.

# *Streptococcus* Group A

Q   What is the optimal management of severe group
    A streptococcal soft tissue infections?

Occasionally, group A streptococci can cause severe potentially life-threatening soft tissue infections; such infections
have been on the rise in recent years. *Early recognition and
institution of appropriate therapy are essential.*

Necrotizing fasciitis (previously called *streptococcal gangrene*)
is a deep-seated infection of the subcutaneous tissue and the
muscle fascia and carries a 10% to 50% mortality. The manifestations of necrotizing fasciitis may be difficult to differentiate from those of cellulitis, which does not usually require
surgical intervention. However, clinical hints such as rapidly
progressing cellulitis in an adequately treated patient, severe
toxicity, and pain disproportionate to the degree of cellulitis
should raise the clinician's suspicion of the possibility of
necrotizing fasciitis. Later during the course of illness, bullae
filled with clear fluid rapidly becoming violaceous in color
and progression to frank cutaneous necrosis often occur.
Whenever there is doubt about the diagnosis, incision and
surgical inspection of the subcutaneous fascia and muscles
should be performed to exclude soft tissue necrosis, which
will require immediate surgical débridement.

Streptococcal myositis is characterized by sudden onset of
pain in the affected muscle, followed by erythema, exquisite

tenderness, edema, decreased motion, fever, and signs of toxicity (e.g., shock); compartment syndrome may also occur. Serum creatine kinase levels are often elevated. Although it is difficult to differentiate necrotizing fasciitis from myositis based on the physical examination alone, the latter has a much higher rate of mortality (80% to 100%) than necrotizing fasciitis. Again, early diagnosis and surgical intervention are essential.

In addition to early surgical intervention, antibiotic treatment should be begun as soon as possible. Although penicillin has traditionally been the drug of choice for severe group A streptococcal infections, there is mounting evidence based on in vitro and in vivo studies that treatment with penicillin therapy alone may be suboptimal.

Clindamycin has several attractive features that make it particularly useful in the treatment of severe group A streptococcal infections, including the following:

1.  Efficacy in killing streptococci even when large numbers are present, a feature not characteristic of penicillin (in vitro and experimental studies suggest a reduction in the efficacy of penicillin when large numbers of streptococci are present ["Eagle effect"]), apparently related to the stationary phase of growth both in vitro and in vivo and to the loss of activity of penicillin against slowly growing organisms

2.  Suppression of the synthesis of bacterial toxins

3.  Facilitation of phagocytosis of group A streptococci by inhibition of M protein synthesis

4.  Suppression of the synthesis of penicillin-binding proteins involved in cell-wall synthesis

5. Suppression of lipopolysaccharide-induced monocyte synthesis of tumor necrosis factor-alpha and, therefore, modulation of the immune response

Although no clinical studies compare clindamycin with or without penicillin with penicillin alone, given the previously mentioned observations and the generally severe nature of streptococcal fasciitis and myositis, combination treatment with clindamycin and penicillin is recommended in such patients.

Other support measures should include aggressive management of shock and multiorgan failure. The value of hyperbaric oxygen therapy remains unproven, and it should never delay surgical intervention. Use of nonsteroidal antiinflammatory agents is discouraged because these agents impair phagocytic function and alter the host's humoral immune response.

## SUGGESTED READINGS

Bisno AL, Stevens DL: Streptococcal infections of skin and soft tissues, *N Engl J Med* 334:240-245, 1996.

Demers B et al: Severe invasive group A streptococcal infections in Ontario, Canada: 1987-1991, *Clin Infect Dis* 16:792-800, 1993.

Forni AL et al: Clinical and microbiological characteristics of severe group A streptococcal infections and streptococcal toxic shock syndrome, *Clin Infect Dis* 21:333-340, 1995.

Stevens DL: Invasive group A *Streptococcus* infections, *Clin Infect Dis* 14:2-11, 1992.

Weiss KA, Laverdiere M: Group A *Streptococcus* invasive infections: a review, *Can J Surg* 40:18-25, 1997.

# Streptococcus pneumoniae

**Q** What is the therapy of choice for pneumococcal pneumonia?

Penicillin had been the standard drug for treatment of pneumococcal pneumonia for many years, given the heretofore predictable susceptibility of *S. pneumoniae* to this antibiotic. Procaine penicillin (600,000 U 2×/day IM) is still appropriate for treatment of penicillin-susceptible (minimum inhibitory concentration less than 0.1 µg/ml for penicillin G) or intermediate (minimum inhibitory concentration between 0.1 µg/ml and 1 µg/ml) strains.

Hospitalized patients are often treated with IV penicillin G 500,000 to 1,000,000 U every 4 hrs; alternatively, a first-generation cephalosporin such as cefazolin 1 g every 8 hrs IV may be used. In bacteremic pneumococcal pneumonia cases, an agent that crosses the blood-brain barrier (e.g., penicillin or a third-generation cephalosporin) should be used preferentially over other agents that do not cross the blood-brain barrier well (e.g., first-generation cephalosporins) because of the possibility of seeding of meninges in this setting.

For outpatients, oral therapy with amoxicillin at a dosage of 500 mg to start, followed by 250 mg every 8 hrs, is an option. Many strains of *S. pneumoniae* have become resistant to erythromycin, tetracyclines, and trimethoprim-sulfamethoxazole, rendering these antibiotics less useful for empiric therapy of infections caused by this organism.

The optimal duration of treatment of pneumococcal pneumonia is unknown. However, most physicians treat pneumococcal pneumonia for 5 to 10 days. For debilitated patients, a regimen of 3 to 5 days of parenteral antibiotic treatment in the hospital, followed by several days of oral therapy not to exceed 5 days after the patient becomes afebrile, has been recommended.

For penicillin-resistant strains (minimum inhibitory concentration 2 µg/ml or more), which are isolated in increasing numbers in recent years, cefotaxime or ceftriaxone is recommended if the minimum inhibitory concentration of cephalosporin for the infecting strain is 8 µg/ml or less. Vancomycin may also be used, particularly when the infecting strain is not fully susceptible to cefotaxime or ceftriaxone.

### SUGGESTED READINGS

Breiman RF et al: Emergence of drug-resistant pneumococcal infections in the United States, *JAMA* 271:1831-1835, 1994.

Friedland IR, McCracken GH Jr: Management of infections caused by antibiotic-resistant *Streptococcus pneumoniae*, *N Engl J Med* 331:377-382, 1994.

Musher DM: Pneumococcal pneumonia including diagnosis and therapy by infection caused by penicillin-resistant strains, *Infect Dis North Am* 5:509-521, 1991.

Musher DM: *Streptococcus pneumoniae*. In Mandell GL, Bennett JE, Dolin R, eds: *Principles and practices of infectious diseases*, ed 4, New York, 1995, Churchill Livingstone.

 For whom is pneumococcal vaccine indicated?

Pneumococcal vaccine is indicated for adults with underlying conditions predisposing to pneumococcal infections or associated with an increased risk of serious disease and its complications.

Specifically, pneumococcal vaccination of patients with the following risk factors is recommended: older age (65 years of age or older); chronic cardiac and pulmonary disease, particularly congestive heart failure; recurrent bronchitis or chronic obstructive lung disease; functional or anatomical asplenia; ulcerative colitis with evidence of hyposplenism on peripheral blood smear; chronic liver disease; alcoholism; diabetes mellitus; chronic renal failure; Hodgkin's disease; chronic lymphocytic leukemia; multiple myeloma; dysglobulinemia; nephrotic syndrome; systemic lupus erythematosus; hemodialysis; primary or metastatic cancer or chemotherapy for malignancies; organ transplantation; HIV infection; cerebrospinal fluid leak (CSF rhinorrhea) secondary to trauma or neurosurgery; and recurrent pneumococcal meningitis. In addition, pneumococcal vaccination should be considered in patients discharged from the hospital after treatment for pneumonia because of an increased risk of this infection during the 3 years after discharge (fivefold higher than those with the initial diagnosis of other infectious diseases).

Note: *Whenever possible, pneumococcal vaccine should be administered before elective splenectomy (at least 10 to 14 days) or planned chemotherapy.*

## SUGGESTED READINGS

ACP Task Force on Adult Immunization and Infectious Diseases Society of America: Pneumococcal infections. In *Guide for adult immunization,* ed 3, Philadelphia, 1994, American College of Physicians.

Gable CB et al: Pneumococcal vaccine; efficacy and associated cost savings, *JAMA* 264:2910-2915, 1990.

Hedlund JU et al: Risk of pneumonia in patients previously treated in hospital for pneumonia, *Lancet* 340:396-397, 1992.

Musher DM: Pneumococcal pneumonia including diagnosis and therapy by infection caused by penicillin-resistant strains, *Infect Dis North Am* 5:509-521, 1991.

Van der Hoeven JG et al: Fatal pneumococcal septic shock in a patient with ulcerative colitis, *Clin Infect Dis* 22:860-861, 1996.

What is the optimal timing of pneumococcal vaccination following a bout of pneumonia?

Immunization at the hospital before discharge would avoid the potential problem with poor compliance and patients not returning for the vaccination. However, many physicians express concern over the efficacy and potential adverse effects of the vaccine when it is given close to the time of diagnosis of pneumococcal pneumonia.

As far as efficacy of vaccination is concerned, it has been suggested that a transient state of unresponsiveness to vaccination might develop in patients for 4 to 6 weeks, but not 8 weeks, following pneumonia. Whether this observation is caused by a transient state of decreased immunological responsiveness or an underlying immune dysfunction predisposing these patients to pneumococcal infection in the first place is unclear.

As far as the risk of adverse reactions is concerned, to date, no study has demonstrated that patients recovering from pneumococcal infections have more severe adverse reactions to pneumococcal vaccine.

It would seem reasonable to delay vaccination of patients until they have fully recovered from their illness (i.e., following discharge from the hospital) and for 8 weeks following their treatment for pneumonia. In those whose medical follow-up is likely to be unpredictable, pneumococcal vaccine may be considered at the time of discharge from the health care facility (author's recommendation).

## SUGGESTED READINGS

Fedson DS, Musher DM: Pneumococcal vaccine. In Plotkin SA, Mortimer EA, eds: *Vaccines,* ed 2, Philadelphia, 1994, WB Saunders.

Hedlund JU et al: Antibody response to pneumococcal vaccine in middle-aged and elderly patients recently treated for pneumonia, *Arch Intern Med* 154:1961-1965, 1994.

# Syphilis

 How should a positive serum rapid plasma reagin (RPR) be interpreted?

RPR and veneral disease research laboratory (VDRL) tests are nontreponemal antibody tests that are often used as a screening test for syphilis. They should be interpreted in conjunction with historical and clinical information regarding the patient. Because false-positive results may be found in those who do not have syphilis (see question in the following section), a reactive RPR or VDRL test should always be confirmed with more specific (but more expensive and labor intensive) treponemal tests such as microhemagglutination assay for *T. pallidum* (MHA-TP) or fluorescent treponemal antibody absorption (FTA-ABS). A reactive RPR and confirmatory test suggest current or previous syphilis infection.

Serum RPR is usually reactive in patients with syphilis, but the percentage of seropositivity varies depending on the stage of the disease: primary syphilis, 80%; secondary syphilis, 99%; and late syphilis, 56%. Titers of RPR are generally reflective of disease activity in early syphilis and are often used to monitor response to therapy.

1. For primary syphilis, a fourfold decline in titers should be expected at 6 months, with eightfold and sixteenfold declines at 12 and 24 months, respectively.

2. For secondary syphilis, eightfold and sixteenfold declines should be observed at 6 and 12 months, respectively.

3. For early latent syphilis, a fourfold decline should not be expected until 12 months.

4. RPR seroreversion to a negative test at 1 year is expected in 50% of patients with an initial episode of only primary syphilis.

## ADDITIONAL CONSIDERATIONS

1. 21% of patients with chronic psychiatric conditions and prior history of syphilis based on a reactive MHA-TP test have a nonreactive serum RPR; therefore serum RPR is *not* a very sensitive test for excluding prior syphilis exposure in this patient population.

2. Even without treatment, serum RPR begins to decline, often reaching relatively low (less than 1:4) titers during the late latent stages and may be negative in neurosyphilis.

3. Results of RPR may vary by less than fourfold dilution on repeat testing of the same sample; therefore such degrees of change in titers between samples drawn at different periods following treatment are usually not considered significant.

### SUGGESTED READINGS

Flores JL: Syphilis: a tale of twisted treponemes, *West J Med* 163:552-559, 1995.

Hook EW III, Marra CM: Acquired syphilis in adults, *N Engl J Med* 326:1060-1069, 1992.

Reeves RR, Pinkofsky HB, Kennedy KK: Unreliability of current screening tests for syphilis in chronic psychiatric patients, *Am J Psychiatry* 153:1487-1488, 1996.

Romanowski B et al: Serologic response to treatment of infectious syphilis, *Ann Intern Med* 114:1005-1009, 1991.

Tramont EC: *Treponema pallidum* (syphilis). In Mandell GL, Bennett JE, Dolin R, eds: *Principles and practices of infectious diseases,* ed 4, New York, 1995, Churchill Livingstone.

What are the potential causes of a false-positive serum RPR or treponemal tests (MHA-TP, FTA-ABS)?

False-positive RPR tests are usually reactive at low dilutions (less than 1:8) and may be associated with a variety of bacterial, viral, and noninfectious conditions.

*Bacterial causes:* pneumococcal pneumonia, scarlet fever, bacterial endocarditis, tuberculosis, mycoplasmal pneumonia, relapsing fever, psittacosis, malaria, rickettsial disease, chancroid, leprosy, lymphogranuloma venereum, leptospirosis, and trypanosomiasis

*Viral causes:* HIV infection, measles, infectious mononucleosis, mumps, viral hepatitis, and vaccinia (vaccination)

*Noninfectious causes:* Pregnancy, chronic liver disease, multiple myeloma, old age, connective tissue disease, multiple blood transfusions, and advanced malignancy

False-positive MHA-TP or FTA-ABS may also occur in the following diseases: Lyme disease, leprosy, relapsing fever, leptospirosis, malaria, infectious mononucleosis, and systemic lupus erythematosus.

### SUGGESTED READING

Hook EW, Marra CM: Acquired syphilis in adults, *N Engl J Med* 326:1060-1069, 1992.

How should an asymptomatic, previously untreated patient with a reactive RPR confirmed by a treponemal test (latent syphilis) be managed?

The primary goal of treatment of latent syphilis is to prevent later development of complications from tertiary disease (e.g., neurosyphilis, aortitis, and gumma). However, up to 10% of patients with late latent (greater than 1 to 2 years' duration) syphilis may have asymptomatic neurosyphilis.

The value of lumbar puncture in all such patients has been questioned and is not routinely recommended except in the following situations: HIV infection, serum RPR or VDRL titer of 1:32 or greater, treatment failure, or planned non-penicillin therapy.

Patients without any of the above risk factors for tertiary syphilis or with one or more of the previously mentioned risk factors but no evidence of neurosyphilis based on spinal fluid examination should be treated with benzathine penicillin G 2.4 million U IM weekly for 3 weeks. Penicillin-allergic patients may be treated with doxycycline 100 mg PO 2×/day for 4 weeks or tetracycline 500 mg PO 4×/day for 4 weeks. Pregnant women with penicillin allergy should undergo desensitization.

### SUGGESTED READINGS

Dowell ME et al: Response of latent syphilis or neurosyphilis to ceftriaxone therapy in persons infected with human immunodeficiency virus, *Am J Med* 93:481-488, 1992.

Flores JL: Syphilis: a tale of twisted treponemes, *West J Med* 163:552-559, 1995.

Rolfs RT: Treatment of syphilis, 1993, *Clin Infect Dis* 20(suppl 1):S23-S38, 1995.

Wiesel J et al: Lumbar puncture in asymptomatic late syphilis: an analysis of the benefits and risks, *Arch Intern Med* 145:465-468, 1985.

# Tick bites

Q

What is the differential diagnosis of erythema around tick bites?

Erythema around tick bites may have several causes, including allergic reaction, cellulitis secondary to bacterial superinfection, and erythema migrans (Lyme disease). Heightened awareness of the public and medical community regarding Lyme disease has led to overdiagnosis of this condition.

Erythema migrans usually develops 3 to 30 days following a tick bite and classically starts as a red macule or papule at the site of the tick bite with expanding margins over several days, often with partial central clearing. The average size of the lesion is 15 cm in diameter, and the area of erythema is usually not associated with symptoms; occasionally burning, pain, pruritus, hyperesthesia, and dysesthesia may occur. Therefore erythematous reactions, particularly when associated with pruritus and occurring within 24 hours following a tick bite, are more likely to be from an allergic reaction than from e. migrans.

Following removal of a tick, in uncomplicated bites, a pruritic erythematous papule or plaque may remain for 1 to 2 weeks. Occasionally a persistent, pruritic, firm and erythematous papule or nodule known as a *tick bite granuloma* develops; intralesional corticosteroids or surgical excision may be required for persistently pruritic lesions.

278

## SUGGESTED READINGS

Asbrink E: Cutaneous manifestations of Lyme borreliosis: clinical defini-
tions and differential diagnoses, *Scand J Infect Dis* 77(suppl):44-50, 1991.
Malane MS et al: Diagnosis of Lyme disease based on dermatologic manifestations, *Ann Intern Med* 114:490-498, 1991.
Wilson B: Ticks. In Mandell GL, Bennett JE, Dolin R, eds: *Principles and practices of infectious diseases,* ed 4, New York, 1995, Churchill Livingstone.

 What is the differential diagnosis of fever following a tick bite?

Several tick-borne diseases are associated with fever: RMSF,
ehrlichiosis, Lyme disease, relapsing fever, Colorado tick
fever, tularemia, and human babesiosis. Although the signs
and symptoms of many of these diseases may be nonspecific,
certain characteristic features may help in distinguishing
them from each other.

RMSF is characterized by pink, blanching macules on the
palms, soles, forearms, legs, and buttocks, which then spread
centripetally to the trunk, neck, and face and within a few
days become petechial.

Ehrlichiosis is usually not associated with a rash or vasculitis
but often presents with leukopenia, absolute lymphocytope-
nia, and rarely inclusions (morulae) in neutrophils, mono-
cytes, and macrophages.

In early Lyme disease, fever (typically low grade and inter-
mittent) may be associated with the characteristic e. migrans
rash, with expanding margins and partial central clearing.

Relapsing fever is characterized by recurrent episodes of fever
(frequently >39° C) lasting an average of 3 days, separated by
afebrile intervals.

Colorado tick fever is associated with a biphasic fever pattern in approximately 50% of cases, starting with a febrile period of 2 to 3 days, followed by an afebrile period lasting 1 to 2 days; it is usually benign and self-limited.

The most common clinical manifestation of tick-borne tularemia is ulceroglandular disease associated with an erythematous, tender papule at the site of the bite that later ulcerates and is usually accompanied by painful regional lymphadenopathy.

Babesiosis is associated with hemolytic anemia of varying degrees and is particularly severe in asplenic patients. The diagnosis is confirmed by the identification of intraerythrocytic parasites in Giemsa-stained peripheral blood smears.

### SUGGESTED READINGS

Doan-Wiggins L: Tick-borne diseases, *Emerg Med Clin Am* 9:303-325, 1991.
Walker DH, Dumler JS: *Ehrlichia chaffeensis* (human ehrlichiosis) and other Ehrlichieae. In Mandell GL, Bennett JE, Dolin R, eds: *Principles and practices of infectious diseases,* ed 4, New York, 1995, Churchill Livingstone.

 Should antibiotic prophylaxis be administered following a tick bite?

Because of the overall low risk of transmission of tick-borne diseases following a tick bite, availability of effective antibiotics for treatment of established disease, and possibility of adverse reactions to antibiotics when used on a large scale, prophylactic antibiotics are generally not considered an important measure in prevention of tick-borne diseases (also see section under "Lyme disease").

## SUGGESTED READINGS

Benenson AS: *Ehrlichiosis: control of communicable diseases manual,* ed 6, Washington, DC, 1995, American Public Health Association.

Benenson AS: *Lyme disease: control of communicable diseases manual,* ed 6, Washington, DC, 1995, American Public Health Association.

Benenson AS: *Rickettsiosis, tickborne: control of communicable diseases manual,* ed 6, Washington, DC, 1995, American Public Health Association.

Benenson AS: *Tularemia: control of communicable diseases manual,* ed 6, Washington, DC, 1995, American Public Health Association.

# Tuberculosis

Q What are the indications for treatment of a positive PPD skin test?

Decision regarding preventive therapy should take into consideration the risk of developing tuberculosis compared with the risk of antituberculous drug toxicity, as well as benefit to society derived from prevention of active tuberculosis. The following persons should be considered for isoniazid preventive therapy:

1. Persons with documented or suspected HIV infection with a skin test reaction 5 mm or greater
2. Persons with a negative tuberculin test (<5 mm) but belonging to groups with high prevalence of tuberculosis infection
3. Close contacts of persons with newly diagnosed tuberculosis with a skin test reaction 5 mm or greater
4. Persons with fibrotic lesion on chest radiograph and a skin test reaction 5 mm or greater
5. Recent tuberculin skin test converters: 10 mm or greater increase within a 2-year period for those younger than 35 years of age or 15 mm or greater increase for those 35 years or older
6. Persons with medical conditions generally considered to be associated with increased risk of tuberculosis and tuberculin reaction 10 mm or greater:
   a. Diabetes mellitus

b. Prolonged therapy with adrenocorticosteroids (>15 mg of daily prednisone); because of the difficulty in predicting long-term corticosteroid requirements and increased risk of isoniazid-associated hepatotoxicity with age, some patients with <15 mg daily prednisone requirement may also be considered for preventive therapy

c. Immunosuppressive therapy

d. Some hematological and reticuloendothelial diseases associated with suppressed cellular immunity (e.g., leukemia or lymphoma)

e. HIV-seronegative injection drug users

f. End-stage renal disease

g. Rapid weight loss or chronic undernutrition (e.g., intestinal bypass surgery for obesity, chronic peptic ulcer disease, chronic malabsorption syndromes, chronic alcoholism, and carcinomas of the oropharynx and upper gastrointestinal tract that interfere with adequate nutritional intake)

h. Postgastrectomy state

7. Persons younger than 35 years of age with skin test 10 mm or greater and belonging to one or more of the following high-incidence groups:

a. Foreign-born persons from high-prevalence countries including many in Latin America, Asia, and Africa

b. Medically under-served low-income populations, including high-risk racial or ethnic minority populations, particularly African Americans, Hispanics, and Native Americans

c. Residents of facilities for long-term care, including correctional and mental institutions and nursing homes

8. Persons with 10 mm or greater tuberculin test reaction and working in facilities in which an individual with active tuberculosis would pose a risk to large numbers of susceptible persons such as correctional and mental

institutions, nursing homes, other health care facilities, schools, and child care facilities

9. Infants and children younger than 4 years of age with a tuberculin skin test reaction 10 mm or greater

10. Children and adolescents with negative tuberculin test (<5 mm) who have been in close contact with an infectious person within the past 3 months; preventive therapy is administered until at least repeat skin testing is performed at 3 months following last exposure

11. Persons younger than 35 years of age with none of the previously mentioned risk factors except a tuberculin skin test reaction 15 mm or greater

Before institution of isoniazid preventive therapy, the following factors should be considered:

1. Exclude bacteriologically positive or radiographically progressive tuberculosis; every person with a significant tuberculin skin test should have a chest radiograph

2. Exclude persons who have been adequately treated for either active tuberculosis or positive skin test in the past

3. Exclude history of prior isoniazid-associated hepatic injury; severe adverse reactions to isoniazid such as drug fever, rash, and arthritis; and concurrent acute or unstable liver disease of any etiology; hepatitis B surface antigenemia is not a contraindication to isoniazid therapy

4. Identify patients for whom special precautions and closer monitoring is indicated:
   a. Age older than 35 years
   b. Concurrent use of other medications with potential interaction
   c. Daily use of alcohol
   d. Previous discontinuation of isoniazid because of possible but not definite related side effects
   e. Current chronic liver disease

   f.  Any condition associated with peripheral neuropathy such as diabetes and alcoholism

   g.  Pregnancy

   h.  Injection drug use

   i.  Female gender, particularly if African-American or Hispanic

SUGGESTED READING

American Thoracic Society: Treatment of tuberculosis and tuberculosis infection in adults and children, *Am J Resp Crit Care Med* 149:1359-1374, 1994.

 Is there a contraindication to tuberculin skin testing during pregnancy, and how should a pregnant woman with a positive tuberculin skin test be managed?

There is no contraindication to the use of tuberculin testing during pregnancy. There is no substantial risk of tuberculosis in women as a result of pregnancy. Therefore preventive therapy is usually delayed until after delivery except in the following circumstances:

1. High-risk medical conditions (see previous section)

2. HIV infection

3. Infection as a result of recent exposure to tuberculosis; isoniazid is generally considered safe during pregnancy

SUGGESTED READING

American Thoracic Society: Treatment of tuberculosis and tuberculosis infection in adults and children, *Am J Resp Crit Care Med* 149:1359-1374, 1994.

# Urinary Tract Infections

 What is the significance of candiduria, and how should it be treated?

In contrast to bacterial UTI, no criteria exist that differentiate between fungal urinary colonization and infection (e.g., pyuria and high colony counts are not helpful). Moreover, upper UTI caused by *Candida* is rare, and its association with asymptomatic or untreated candiduria is unclear. Diabetes mellitus, obstructive uropathy, and renal transplantation have been *suggested* to be risk factors for the progression of uncomplicated candiduria to more serious disease, but well-designed scientific studies are lacking.

Indications for treatment of asymptomatic candiduria are unclear. Removal of predisposing factors (e.g., Foley catheter, antibiotics, and immunosuppressants) should be considered whenever possible. Up to 65% of patients may have clearance of candiduria in the absence of specific therapy. Treatment should be considered for patients with diabetes, obstructive uropathy, and immunocompromised status.

Treatment options include the following:

1.  Fluconazole 200 mg followed by 100 mg/day for 4 days (not recommended for *C. torulopsis)*

2.  Amphotericin B continuous bladder irrigation 50 mg/L of sterile water at 42 ml/hr for 48 hrs

**286**

3. Amphotericin B 10 to 30 mg in 250 to 400 ml $D_5W$ via urinary catheter; cross-clamp the catheter for "as long as possible" 4×/day for up to 15 days (in the author's experience, sterile water instead of $D_5W$ may be used with clamping of the catheter for about 1 hr each time, for 1 week)

4. Amphotericin B IV 0.3 mg/kg single dose

### SUGGESTED READINGS

Carr M, Dismukes WE: Antifungal drugs. In Gorbach SL, Bartlett JG, Blacklow NR, eds: *Infectious diseases,* Philadelphia, 1992, WB Saunders.

Fan-Havard P et al: Oral fluconazole versus amphotericin B bladder irrigation for treatment of candidal funguria, *Clin Infect Dis* 21:960-965, 1995.

Gubbins PO, Piscitelli SC, Danziger LH: Candidal urinary tract infections: a comprehensive review of their diagnosis and management, *Pharmacotherapy* 13:110-127, 1993.

Leu HS, Huang CT: Clearance of funguria with short-course antifungal regimens: a prospective randomized, controlled study, *Clin Infect Dis* 20:1152-1157, 1995.

Wong-Beringer A, Jacobs RA, Guglielmo BJ: Treatment of funguria, *JAMA* 267:2780-2785, 1992.

 What is the significance of coagulase-negative *Staphylococcus* grown from urine cultures, and how should it be treated?

Two major causes of coagulase-negative staphylococcal UTI are *Staphylococcus saprophyticus* and *S. epidermidis. S. saprophyticus* affects primarily sexually active healthy women 16 to 35 years old; is symptomatic in 90% of cases; and usually responds to ampicillin, cephalosporins, and quinolones. It is invariably resistant to nalidixic acid, with therapeutic failure with nitrofurantoin and sulfonamide reported. It is a contaminant from urine in only 5% of the cases.

*S. epidermidis* rarely causes UTI. It is found almost exclusively in the urine of hospitalized patients with indwelling urinary catheter or recent urinary tract surgery, renal transplantation, neurogenic bladder, stones, or obstruction. It is associated with pyuria and clinically significant UTI in only 10% of cases (i.e., asymptomatic in 90%), affects primarily older patients (older than 50 years old), and affects women and men equally. The organism is usually resistant to multiple antibiotics; antibiotic selection when necessary should be based on in vitro susceptibility test results.

### SUGGESTED READINGS

Archer GL: *Staphylococcus epidermidis* and other coagulase-negative staphylococci. In Mandell GL, Bennett JE, Dolin R, eds: *Principles and practices of infectious diseases,* ed 4, New York, 1995, Churchill Livingstone.

Hovelius B, Mardh PA: *Staphylococcus saprophyticus* as a common cause of urinary tract infection, *Rev Infect Dis* 6:328-337, 1984.

 When should asymptomatic bacteriuria be treated?

Treatment of asymptomatic bacteriuria is recommended for children and during pregnancy. In older adults, asymptomatic bacteriuria is common and usually requires no therapy except under the following circumstances: genitourinary procedures, implantation of a prosthetic device, urinary obstruction when drainage procedure is not practical, and when major surgery is planned.

Note: *1. Treatment of institutionalized elderly patients for asymptomatic bacteriuria does not significantly decrease morbidity or mortality but may result in increased adverse effects secondary to antibiotics and emergence of antimicrobial resistance.*

*2. Pyuria is common in elderly institutionalized patients and, by itself, is not a useful discriminator for selection of asymptomatic subjects for antimicrobial therapy.*

## SUGGESTED READINGS

Childs SJ, Egan RJ: Bacteriuria and urinary infections in the elderly, *Urol Clin North Am* 23:43-54, 1996.

Nicolle LE: Urinary tract infection in the institutionalized elderly, *Infect Dis Clin Pract* 1:68-71, 1992.

Sobel JD, Kaye D: Urinary tract infections. In Mandell GL, Bennett JE, Dolin R, eds: *Principles and practices of infectious diseases,* ed 4, New York, 1995, Churchill Livingstone.

 How should enterococcal UTIs be treated?

UTIs caused by enterococci usually respond to single-drug therapy such as ampicillin, penicillin G, or vancomycin. Ureidopenicillins (e.g., piperacillin and mezlocillin) should also be effective but are more expensive. Nitrofurantoin may be used for enterococcal cystitis in the absence of renal insufficiency. Quinolones (e.g., ciprofloxacin and ofloxacin) may be used against some enterococcal UTIs, but increasing resistance limits their effectiveness (see the following section).

Note: *Aminoglycosides (as single agent), cephalosporins, trimethoprim-sulfamethoxazole, carbenicillin, ticarcillin, and oxacillin/nafcillin are not recommended for treatment of enterococcal infections.*

## SUGGESTED READINGS

Moellering RC: *Enterococcus* species, *Streptococcus bovis,* and *Leuconostoc* species. In Mandell GL, Bennett JE, Dolin R, eds: *Principles and practices of infectious diseases,* ed 4, New York, 1995, Churchill Livingstone.

Murray BE: The life and times of the *Enterococcus, Clin Microbiol Rev* 3:46-65, 1990.

Tailor SA, Bailey EM, Rybak MJ: *Enterococcus*, an emerging pathogen, *Ann Pharmacother* 27:1231-1242, 1993.

 What are the limitations of quinolones (e.g., ciprofloxacin) in the treatment of UTIs?

Ciprofloxacin has excellent activity in vitro against most aerobic gram-negative bacilli causing UTIs (e.g., *E. coli, Enterobacter* sp., *P. aeruginosa, Serratia* sp.) but is significantly less active against many staphylococci (see pp. 260-261), streptococcal species, and enterococci.

Quinolones are not recommended in children or for pregnant or nursing women because of the finding of cartilage erosions and arthropathies in weight-bearing joints of experimental animals. These drugs should also be used with caution in patients with underlying seizure disorder.

Coadministration of quinolones with theophylline or warfarin can lead to theophylline toxicity and increased prothrombin time, respectively. Aluminum-, magnesium-, and to a lesser extent calcium-containing antacids severely reduce gastrointestinal absorption of quinolones. In certain patients with cancer, use of ciprofloxacin has been associated with nephrotoxicity.

### SUGGESTED READINGS

Hendershot EF: Fluoroquinolones, *Infec Dis Clin North Am* 9:715-730, 1995.
Lo WK et al: Ciprofloxacin-induced nephrotoxicity in patients with cancer, *Arch Intern Med* 153:1258-1262, 1993.
Mott FE, Murphy S, Hunt V: Ciprofloxacin and warfarin, *Ann Intern Med* 111:542-543, 1989.

## STIMULATING QUESTION

Why do patients with ileal urinary conduit get frequent UTIs?

Up to 84% of patients undergoing urinary diversion by ileal conduit develop bacteriuria caused by a variety of organisms (e.g., *E. coli, Candida* sp., *Pseudomonas* sp., and *Streptococcus* sp.), with 14% of patients developing pyelonephritis. The mucus, produced by the goblet cells within the ileal conduit, forms a dense biofilm that entraps organisms. This process, although preventing the attachment of organisms to the columnar cell surface of the conduit, may in the absence of ileo-ureteral valve facilitate the reflux of bacteria in the mucous biofilm into the kidneys. In addition, chronic exposure of the ileal mucosa to urine is thought to lead to severe depletion of lymphoid elements and atrophy of Peyer's patches, thus increasing the risk of infection by pathogenic bacteria.

### SUGGESTED READINGS

Bruce AW et al: Bacterial adherence in the human ileal conduit: a morphological and bacteriological study, *J Urol* 132:184-187, 1984.
Tapper D, Folkman J: Lymphoid depletion in ileal loops: mechanism and clinical implication, *J Pediatr Surg* 11:871-880, 1976.

# Vancomycin

 Is vancomycin ototoxic or nephrotoxic?

Although vancomycin was originally thought to be ototoxic and nephrotoxic, recent animal studies have not been able to confirm either one of these adverse reactions when vancomycin is administered alone.

Clinically, vancomycin-associated ototoxicity has been rare in patients with normal renal function receiving usual doses of the drug. Many patients with vancomycin-associated ototoxicity have had kidney dysfunction or underlying auditory dysfunction. Furthermore, frequent concurrent or recent treatment with other well-known ototoxic drugs such as aminoglycosides makes it difficult to differentiate the relative contribution of vancomycin to the ototoxicity. Of note, animal studies have found augmentation of gentamicin-associated ototoxicity in the presence of vancomycin. However, it is unclear at what vancomycin serum concentrations vancomycin might enhance ototoxicity of other drugs in patients.

Similar to ototoxicity, vancomycin as a cause of nephrotoxicity when used alone has been uncommon, despite the widespread reputation to the contrary. The reported incidence of vancomycin-related nephrotoxicity has been usually between 5% and 7% in trials that controlled for potentially confounding factors. Interestingly, these rates of renal insufficiency have also been observed in certain antibiotics (e.g., cefamandole and penicillin) not considered nephrotoxic. Although

**292**

trough serum concentrations of vancomycin greater than or equal to 10 µg/ml have been reported to be associated with renal dysfunction, it is not at all clear whether such concentrations actually cause nephrotoxicity or whether they are simply a reflection of poor clearance of vancomycin by the kidneys.

Combination therapy with vancomycin and aminoglycoside has been reported to potentiate the nephrotoxicity of aminoglycosides in both animal models and in humans, particularly when treatment duration is greater than 3 weeks; the latter observation has not been consistently demonstrated. Again, the role of vancomycin serum levels in preventing this complication has not been elucidated.

In summary, based on current clinical data, when used alone, vancomycin appears to be only weakly ototoxic or nephrotoxic, if at all.

### SUGGESTED READINGS

Cantu TG, Yamanaka-Yuen NA, Lietman PS: Serum vancomycin concentrations: reappraisal of their clinical value, *Clin Infect Dis* 18:533-543, 1994.

Cunha BA: Vancomycin, *Med Clin North Am* 79:817-831, 1995.

Goldstein E et al: Are serum levels of vancomycin useful in the first week of therapy? *Mo Med* 92:596-599, 1995.

Moellering RC Jr: Monitoring serum vancomycin levels: climbing the mountain because it is there? *Clin Infect Dis* 18:544-546, 1994 (editorial).

 In what clinical situations is measurement of vancomycin serum concentrations indicated?

In light of the uncertainties regarding the potential ototoxicity and nephrotoxicities of vancomycin and the difficulties in determining blood/drug concentrations predictive of such complications (see previous section), measurement of vancomycin levels is not routinely recommended when used in usual doses and corrected for renal insufficiency.

Because trough vancomycin levels are predictive of peak values, measurement of trough levels seems reasonable in the following situations:

1.   Patients receiving vancomycin/aminoglycoside combinations, particularly when the duration of therapy exceeds 3 weeks

2.   Dialysis patients receiving infrequent doses of vancomycin to ensure constant therapeutic levels of vancomycin

3.   Patients with high total body weight (e.g., very obese patients) or volume of distribution (e.g., patients with burns or ascites) because of the possibility of subtherapeutic levels with normal dosage

4.   Patients requiring higher-than-usual doses of vancomycin (e.g., for meningitis)

5.   Patients with rapidly changing renal function

In addition, monitoring CSF vancomycin levels is reasonable when it is used for treatment of meningitis because of reported treatment failures when vancomycin CSF levels are inadequate.

### SUGGESTED READINGS

Cunha BA: Vancomycin, *Med Clin North Am* 79:817-831, 1995.
Kucers A, Bennett N McK: *The use of antibiotics,* Philadelphia, 1987, JB Lippincott.
Moellering RC Jr: Monitoring serum vancomycin levels: climbing the mountain because it is there? *Clin Infect Dis* 18:544-546, 1994 (editorial).

How should serum vancomycin levels be interpreted?

Because of the presence of good correlation between peak and trough serum vancomycin levels and the potential for high variability in levels when not obtained at 2 hours postinfusion, measurement of peak levels is not recommended.

Even with trough vancomycin levels, as previously discussed (see question regarding ototoxicity and nephrotoxicity), it is not at all clear that their measurement will necessarily decrease the risk of toxicity from vancomycin. When toxicity has been associated with vancomycin, the measured trough serum concentrations have usually been greater than 20 µg/ml. Therefore in situations in which vancomycin is not expected to clear normally or when a higher-than-usual dose (adults, 1 g IV every 12 hrs) is administered, it is reasonable to attempt to maintain serum trough levels less than 20 µg/ml.

Although the value of measurement of serum levels of vancomycin in determining its clinical efficacy has not been extensively studied, studies to date suggest that maintenance of serum trough levels at or above 10 µg/ml may be important therapeutically.

For these reasons, when measurement of vancomycin trough levels appear to be indicated, serum concentrations between 10 and 20 µg/ml should be achieved; previously recommended trough levels less than 10 µg/ml seem too restrictive.

SUGGESTED READINGS

Moellering RC Jr: Monitoring serum vancomycin levels: climbing the mountain because it is there? *Clin Infect Dis* 18:544-546, 1994 (editorial).

Mulhern JG et al: Trough serum vancomycin levels predict the relapse of gram-positive peritonitis in peritoneal dialysis patients, *Am J Kidney Dis* 25:611-615, 1995.

Saunders NJ: Why monitor peak vancomycin concentrations? *Lancet* 344:1748-1750, 1994.

Zimmermann AE, Katona BG, Plaisance KI: Association of vancomycin serum concentrations with outcomes in patients with gram-positive bacteremia, *Pharmacotherapy* 15:85-91, 1995.

 How should the "red man's" or "red neck" reaction from vancomycin infusion be prevented or managed?

Red man, or red neck, reaction is characterized by pruritus and intense erythema involving the face, neck, upper body, back, and upper extremities and is thought to occur secondary to nonimmunologically mediated release of histamine from mast cells. This reaction often occurs when IV vancomycin is given rapidly (e.g., 1-g dose given over less than 1 hr). Longer infusion times and pretreatment with antihistamines such as diphenhydramine or hydroxyzine are effective in preventing the syndrome.

When red man's syndrome does occur, temporary discontinuation of infusion and administration of an antihistamine such as diphenhydramine, IV fluids (if hypotension is present), and less frequently corticosteroids are recommended. Because this reaction is not truly allergic in origin, vancomycin may be readministered with proper premedication and infusion time.

### SUGGESTED READINGS

Cunha BA: Vancomycin, *Med Clin North Am* 79:817-831, 1995.

Kucers A, Bennett N McK: *The use of antibiotics*, Philadelphia, 1987, JB Lippincott.

How should vancomycin dose be adjusted in renal insufficiency?

The usual dose of IV vancomycin in patients with normal renal function is 1 g every 12 hrs or 500 mg every 6 hrs. Because vancomycin is eliminated by the kidneys via glomerular filtration, its serum half-life becomes prolonged in renal insufficiency and may therefore be administered less frequently as follows:

Creatinine clearance >50 ml/min: 1 g every 12 to 24 hrs
Creatinine clearance >10 ml/min but <50 ml/min: 1 g every 1 to 4 days
Creatinine clearance less than 10 ml/min: 1 g every 4 to 7 days

Hemodialysis and peritoneal dialysis patients are typically administered vancomycin 1 g every week because this antibiotic is not removed significantly by usual dialysis methods (except when high-flux dialysis membranes are used). However, because of the potential for prolonged subtherapeutic serum concentrations in seriously ill patients with renal insufficiency, measurement of serum trough levels at least initially is suggested. In peritoneal dialysis patients with gram-positive peritonitis and in whom vancomycin trough levels cannot be measured in a timely manner, dosing of vancomycin every 5 days has been recommended by some authors.

### SUGGESTED READINGS

Cunha BA: Vancomycin, *Med Clin North Am* 79:817-831, 1995.
Mulhern JG et al: Trough serum vancomycin levels predict the relapse of gram-positive peritonitis in peritoneal dialysis patients, *Am J Kidney Dis* 25:611-615, 1995.
Sanford JP, Gilbert DN, Sande MA: *Guide to antimicrobial therapy,* ed 26, Dallas, 1996, Antimicrobial Therapy.

# Varicella (Chicken Pox)

 How should exposure of susceptible persons to varicella be managed?

The decision to use VZIG depends on the likelihood that a given exposure is "significant" (i.e., will result in infection), that the exposed individual will develop complications of varicella if infected, and that the individual is susceptible to varicella.

"Significant" exposure includes residence in the same household; face-to-face indoor play; stay in the same hospital room; face-to-face contact with an infectious staff member or patient; in-hospital visit by a potentially contagious person; and in the case of a newborn infant, onset of varicella in the mother 5 days or less before delivery or within 48 hours after delivery; VZIG is not indicated if the mother has zoster. Patients are considered contagious from 1 to 2 days before and as long as 5 days after the onset of rash in immunocompetent patients, probably longer in immunocompromised persons.

VZIG (125 U/10 kg of body weight, maximum 625 U) should be given by IM (not IV) injection within 48 hrs of and not more than 96 hrs after exposure; it is expensive (approximately $400.00 for an average adult) and provides only temporary protection.

VZIG candidates include immunocompromised patients (children and adults, including those with HIV infection) without

**298**

history of chicken pox, susceptible pregnant women, bone marrow recipients (regardless of history of varicella or zoster before transplant and without history of varicella or zoster following transplant), newborn infants whose mothers have onset of chicken pox within 5 days before delivery or within 2 days after delivery, hospitalized premature infants (less than 28 weeks, gestation) whose mothers have no history of chicken pox, and hospitalized premature infants (less than 28 weeks' gestation or 1000 g or less) regardless of maternal history. Neonates born to mothers who have signs and symptoms of varicella within 5 days preceding or 2 days after delivery should also receive VZIG regardless of whether the mother received VZIG. VZIG may prolong the incubation period of varicella from 10 to 21 days to 28 days or greater. The duration for which VZIG recipients are protected against chicken pox is unknown, but a recipient exposed to varicella more than 3 weeks after the administration of VZIG should receive a repeat dose. Patients receiving monthly treatments of high-dose IV immunoglobulin are probably protected and may not require VZIG if the last dose was given 3 weeks or less before exposure to wild-type VZV.

Because of the availability of effective therapy (e.g., acyclovir), administration of VZIG in normal healthy susceptible adults is not routinely recommended.

## SUGGESTED READINGS

American Academy of Pediatrics: Varicella-zoster infections. In Peter G, ed: *1994 Red Book: report of the Committee on Infectious Diseases,* ed 23, Elk Grove Village, Ill, 1994, American Academy of Pediatrics.

American Academy of Pediatrics: Varicella-zoster infections. In Peter G, ed: *1997 Red Book: report of the Committee on Infectious Diseases,* ed 24, Elk Grove Village, Ill, 1997, American Academy of Pediatrics.

Centers for Disease Control and Prevention: Prevention of varicella; recommendations of the Advisory Committee on Immunization Practices (ACIP), *MMWR* (suppl) 45(RR-11):1-36, 1996.

How should chicken pox in immunocompetent hosts be treated?

Oral acyclovir is not recommended routinely for treatment of uncomplicated varicella in otherwise healthy children (except secondary household cases in which the disease is usually more severe) because of its marginal therapeutic effect, cost of the drug, and impracticality of initiating the drug in the first 24 hrs of illness. If oral acyclovir is used in children, it should be begun within 24 hrs of the onset of rash at a daily dose of 80 mg/kg in four divided doses for 5 days (maximum 3200 mg/day).

Oral acyclovir should be considered for those older than 12 years of age, adults, persons with chronic cutaneous or pulmonary disorders, and those receiving chronic salicylate therapy. The usual dose is 800 mg 5×/day for 5 days, assuming normal renal function.

Because of its life-threatening nature, varicella pneumonia (particularly in pregnant women) should be treated with IV acyclovir at a dosage of 10 mg/kg every 8 hrs.

Children with varicella should not receive salicylates because their administration increases the risk of subsequent Reye's syndrome.

### SUGGESTED READINGS

American Academy of Pediatrics: Varicella-zoster infections. In Peter G, ed: *1994 Red Book: report of the Committee on Infectious Diseases*, ed 23, Elk Grove Village, Ill, 1994, American Academy of Pediatrics.

American Academy of Pediatrics: Varicella-zoster infections. In Peter G, ed: *1997 Red Book: report of the Committee on Infectious Diseases*, ed 24, Elk Grove Village, Ill, 1997, American Academy of Pediatrics.

Whitley RJ, Straus SE: Therapy for varicella-zoster virus infections: where do we stand? *Infect Dis Clin Pract* 2:100-108, 1993.

How should the varicella vaccine be used?

The American Academy of Pediatrics recommends a single dose of the vaccine (subcutaneous) for healthy children 12 to 18 months of age if there is no history of varicella. Between 18 months and 13 years, a single dose is also recommended for children who are not already immunized and who have no history of varicella. Varicella vaccine may be given simultaneously with the measles-mumps-rubella (MMR) vaccine, as long as different sites and syringes are used. If the MMR and varicella vaccines are not given simultaneously, a month interval between vaccines is recommended.

Unimmunized adolescents 13 years of age or older and adults who have no history of varicella should receive two doses 4 to 8 weeks apart. Postimmunization serological evaluation is not routinely recommended among these individuals (99% seroconversion rate after two doses), with the possible exception of health care workers who may pose a nosocomial risk if they fail to respond adequately. Inadvertent immunization of seropositive individuals is not associated with an increased risk of side effects.

Varicella vaccine is a live-attenuated vaccine. It is contraindicated in pregnancy and in immunocompromised patients with any type of humoral or cell-mediated deficiency, including transplant recipients, HIV-infected patients, patients with malignancies, or those receiving chemotherapy. Under protocol, the vaccine may be used in children 1 to 17 years old who have acute lymphocytic leukemia if they have been in remission for at least 1 year. Women of childbearing age should be counseled against pregnancy for at least 1 month following immunization. Children treated with the equivalent of prednisone 2 mg/kg or greater per day should not be immunized until steroid therapy has been discontinued for at least 1 month. Salicylate therapy should be avoided for 1 month, if possible, following immunization because of the theoretical association of Reye's syndrome with salicylates and varicella immunization.

### SUGGESTED READINGS

American Academy of Pediatrics: Varicella-zoster infections. In Peter G, ed: *1997 Red Book: report of the Committee on Infectious Diseases,* ed 24, Elk Grove Village, Ill, 1997, American Academy of Pediatrics.

Gershon AA et al: Varicella vaccine: the American experience, *J Infect Dis* 166(suppl 1):S63-S68, 1992.

Meissner HC: Varicella vaccine: the first licensed herpes vaccine, *Infect Dis Clin Pract* 5:424-427, 1996.

Who should be considered susceptible to varicella (chicken pox)?

Persons with a history of varicella are usually considered immune; however, those without such a history may also be immune. In evaluating whether a person without a history of varicella is likely to be susceptible, the following may be helpful: (1) history of varicella in siblings (particularly younger siblings); (2) attendance in urban school; (3) previous exposure to patients with chicken pox or zoster without developing disease. When in doubt, serological testing (e.g., FAMA, LA, or ELISA) for detection of varicella antibody (IgG) is helpful in determining the immune status.

Symptomatic reinfection is rare in healthy persons, but asymptomatic reinfection can occur. Asymptomatic primary infection is uncommon.

## SUGGESTED READINGS

American Academy of Pediatrics: Varicella-zoster infections. In Peter G, ed: *1997 Red Book: report of the Committee on Infectious Diseases,* ed 24, Elk Grove Village, Ill, 1997, American Academy of Pediatrics.

Arvin AM: Immune responses to varicella-zoster virus, *Infect Dis Clin North Am* 10:529-570, 1996.

# Index

Cytomegalovirus (CMV), 77-83
  in body fluids, 80
  culture of, from bronchoalveolar
    lavage, 82-83
  exposure to, in pregnancy, 81
  isolation of, from blood or urine,
    interpretation of, 82
  transmission of, 78-80
Cytomegalovirus (CMV)-specific IgG
    antibody tests, interpreta-
    tion of, 77-78

**D**

Decubitus ulcers
  cellulitis associated with, 53-54
  osteomyelitis associated with
    diagnosis of, 227-228
    management of, 228
Dental procedures, endocarditis pro-
    phylaxis for, 90
Diabetes mellitus, cellulitis associated
    with, 54
Diarrhea
  *Campylobacter*-associated, treatment
    of, 34-35
  *Clostridium difficile*-associated, 75-76
  cryptosporidial, 111
  traveler's
    ciprofloxacin in treatment/pre-
      vention of, 69
    prevention and treatment of,
      107-108
Didanosine, ciprofloxacin interaction
    with, 71
Direct fluorescent antibody in Legion-
    naires' pneumonia diagno-
    sis, 179
Dissecting cellulitis of scalp, 54
Diverticulitis, 84-86
DNA probe/hybridization tests in
    Legionnaires' pneumonia
    diagnosis, 179
Dog bite
  cellulitis from, 55
    management of, 21
  management of, 19-20
Doxycycline for malaria prophylaxis
  adult dosage regimen for, 201
  contraindications for, 202
  countries indicated for, 200
  side effects of, 202

Drainage in bacterial arthritis man-
    agement, 5-6
Drug(s)
  injection use of, HIV transmission
    risk and, 143
  interactions of ciprofloxacin with,
    70-71

**E**

Eastern equine encephalitis virus,
    meningitis from, 205-206
Ehrlichiosis, 279
Encephalitis, HSV, management/pre-
    vention of, 132
Encephalitis viruses, meningitis from,
    205-206
Endocarditis, 87-99
  cardiac conditions requiring pro-
    phylaxis for, 87-89
  enterococcal, antibiotics for,
    100-101
  prophylaxis for, 90-99
    antibiotics for, 94-99
    contraindications to, 92-94
    indications for, 90-91
Enteritis, *Campylobacter,* postinfec-
    tious complications of, 36
*Enterobacter,* respiratory tract infec-
    tions from, treatment of,
    187-188
Enterococcus, 100-102
  urinary tract infections from, treat-
    ment of, 289
Enterovirus, meningitis from, 204-205
Epstein-Barr virus (EBV), 103-106
  mononucleosis from, management
    of, 105
  serological test interpretation for,
    103
*Erysipelothrix rhusiopathiae,* cellulitis
    from, 55
Erythema around tick bites, differen-
    tial diagnosis of, 278
Erythema migrans
  following tick bites, 278
  risk of Lyme disease transmission
    from patient with, 192
Erythromycin
  for *Campylobacter*-associated diar-
    rhea, 35

Erythromycin—*cont'd*
for Legionnaires' pneumonia, 180-181
Esophagus, candidiasis of, treatment of, 43-44

**F**

Famciclovir for herpes zoster, 136
Fasciitis, necrotizing, management of, 266
Fatigue, chronic, EBV antibody testing in, 104
Fever blisters, kissing safety and, 134-135
Fever following tick bite, differential diagnosis of, 279-280
Fluconazole (Diflucan)
for candidal vulvovaginitis, 40-41
for esophageal candidiasis, 44
for oral candidiasis, 42-43
for urinary tract infection, 286
Fluorescent treponemal antibody absorption (FTA-ABS)
false-positive, causes of, 276
positive, interpretation of, 274-275
Fluoroquinolones
adverse effects of, 65-67
resistance to, 64

**G**

Gangrene, streptococcal, management of, 266
Gastroenteritis, 107-111
*Blastocystis hominis,* 109
cryptosporidial, 111
*Salmonella,* 109-110
traveler's diarrhea as, 107-108
Gastrointestinal tract
adverse effects of fluoroquinolones on, 65
endocarditis prophylaxis for, 90-91
Genital herpes
acyclovir dosage for, 1
management/prevention of, 130-131
spermicides in preventing transmission of, 135
Genitourinary tract, endocarditis prophylaxis for, 91
Gentamicin for endocarditis prophylaxis, 96

Glyburide, ciprofloxacin interaction with, 71
Gonococcal arthritis, management of, 5-6
Granuloma
swimming pool, treatment of, 221-222
tick bite, 278
Guillain-Barré syndrome
following *Campylobacter jejuni* infections, 36
influenza vaccine for person with history of, 173-174

**H**

*Haemophilus influenzae*
lower respiratory tract infections from, treatment of, 184
pharyngitis and, 242
*Haemophilus influenzae* type B meningitis, chemoprophylaxis for, 208-209
Hearing, adverse effects of fluoroquinolones on, 66
Heart conditions, bacterial endocarditis prophylaxis for, 87-89
Hematologic system, adverse effects of fluoroquinolones on, 67
Hemophiliacs, HIV transmission risk in, 143
Hepatitis A, 112-116
prophylaxis for, 112-114
transmission of, 115
Hepatitis B, 117-119
carrier of, school for, 119
needlestick exposure to, evaluation/prophylaxis following, 213, 214t
serological tests for, 117
testing for, after human bite, 22
vaccination for, indications for, 118-119
Hepatitis C, 120-128
antibody for, positive
in asymptomatic person, interpretation of, 120-121
patient with, management of, 122-123
needlestick exposure to, evaluation/prophylaxis following, 214

# NOTES

# NOTES

# NOTES

# NOTES